Take Charge
of Your
Health

Books by Hans Diehl and Aileen Ludington

Dynamic Living
Dynamic Living Workbook
Health Power
Reversing High Blood Pressure Naturally
Reversing Obesity Naturally
Feeling Fit
Healthy Beginnings DVD
Diet for a New Century (audio)
CHIP (20-video series)

To order, call 1-800-765-6955.
Visit us at *www.reviewandherald.com* for information on other Review and Herald products.

Take Charge
of Your
Health

AILEEN LUDINGTON, MD

HANS DIEHL, DrHSc, MPH

REVIEW AND HERALD® PUBLISHING ASSOCIATION
Since 1861 | www.reviewandherald.com

The authors assume full responsibility for the accuracy of all
facts and quotations as cited in this book.

Texts credited to Clear Word are from *The Clear Word,*
copyright © 1994 by Jack J. Blanco.
Texts credited to NIV are from the *Holy Bible, New
International Version.* Copyright © 1973, 1978, 1984, International
Bible Society. Used by permission of Zondervan Bible Publishers.
Bible texts credited to RSV are from the Revised Standard
Version of the Bible, copyright © 1946, 1952, 1971, by the
Division of Christian Education of the National Council of the
Churches of Christ in the U.S.A. Used by permission.

This book was
Edited by Jeannette R. Johnson
Copyedited by Jocelyn Fay and James Cavil
Designed by Madelyn Ruiz
Electronic makeup by Shirley M. Bolivar
Cover photos: PhotoDisc
Typeset: Bembo 11/13

PRINTED IN U.S.A.

12 11 10 09   10 9 8 7

R&H Cataloging Service
Ludington, Aileen, 1924-
    Life choices: the incredible power of the body to heal itself,
by Aileen Ludington and Hans Diehl.

    1. Health.   2. Health self-care.   I. Diehl, Hans, 1946-
II. Title

613.7
Adapted from *Dynamic Living, Health Power,* and *Feeling Fit*

ISBN 978-0-8280-1559-2

CONTENTS

About This Book . . .

The stories in this book are about people who made lifestyle and medication changes WITH the guidance of qualified health professionals. We urge you to do the same.

Many of the names and some of the places mentioned have been changed to protect the privacy of those involved.

To avoid duplication, all lifestyle changes made are not enumerated in each story. Please refer to the Coda at the back of the book. It summarizes the guiding principles of lifestyle medicine that promote optimum health and that reverse many diseases.

The stories involving community seminars are largely drawn from CHIP (Coronary Health Improvement Project), a 40-hour health education program developed by Dr. Hans Diehl. For more information, call 909-796-7676. The stories involving time spent in a "live-in health center" are mostly experiences Dr. Aileen Ludington recorded while she was a physician at the NEWSTART Lifestyle Center at Weimar Institute, Weimar, CA 95736. For more information, call 800-525-9192.

About the Authors . . .

Aileen Ludington, M.D., is an internationally known health educator and author. She spent seven years as medical adviser for the *Westbrook Hospital* television series. Her six books on health have sold more than a half million copies and have been translated into several languages. In 1999 Dr. Ludington was chosen Woman of the Year by Loma Linda University's medical auxiliary and lives in Paradise, California.

Hans Diehl, Dr.H.Sc., M.P.H., C.S.N., F.A.C.N., is the founder and director of the Lifestyle Medicine Institute in Loma Linda, California. His book *Health Power* (Vida Dinámica), coauthored with Aileen Ludington, M.D., has more than 1.5 million copies in 16 languages in circulation. Diehl was chosen one of America's 20 superheroes in the health movement. He lives with his wife, Dr. Lily Diehl, in Loma Linda, California.

The Setting:
The Gun and the Bible

I looked over the small group in the waiting room. "Hattie Hammond?"

A small lump of a woman struggled to get up from her chair. She looked like Mother Time—old, weak, tottering on her cane. As I helped her into my office, I wondered about her expectations. Did she think our health center offered nursing home care? She sat down, locked her eyes into mine, and launched into her story.

DOCTORS SHOULD REALIZE PEOPLE DON'T FEEL OLD, THEY JUST LOOK THAT WAY.

"So I lay there with a gun to my head and a Bible on my heart. I was totally miserable, and I had no more money for doctors or medicines. Would I live, or would I die? I decided to sell my house and come here." Her eyes burned with intensity. "So you see, this place is my last hope—my desperation station."

What an opener! I stared at her, wondering how to proceed. She anticipated my question and handed me a neatly printed list of her medical problems—all 12 of them, all of them serious. Her gait may have been unsteady, but her 84-year-old mind was as keen as mine. I wrote the 12 symptoms on her chart and introduced her to the program she would be following.

Four weeks later, at graduation time, she surprised me once more by handing me a progress report on her 12 problems:

"BEFORE"	"AFTER"
1. Hypoglycemic shakes	No hypoglycemia
2. Hypertension	Blood pressure coming down
3. Obesity	Lost 10 pounds
4. Swollen legs	No more swelling
5. Painful joints	No pain in any joint
6. Constipation	No constipation
7. Urinary frequency	Get up only once at night
8. Can't walk	Can walk one-half mile
9. Insomnia	Sleep well
10. Chest congestion and chronic cough	Congestion and cough gone
11. Painful feet	No pain in feet
12. Depressed	No depression

Hattie smiled happily. "After 10 years of treatments and $50,000," she said, "I never felt so good as I did after only a few days here. I praise God for this health center. I can go to church again. I'm canceling the convalescent home—I'm going house hunting!"

∞

Is this story unique? More dramatic than most, perhaps, but not that unusual. It's almost never too late to significantly improve one's health by making some relatively simple lifestyle changes.

What actually happened to Hattie at the health center? What did she do? What did we do? Was there some special magic involved in her transformation?

This book is about the incredible power of the

body to heal itself, given proper attention to lifestyle factors. We will share with you, step by step, true story after true story, how most of the common diseases, ailments, and disabilities people suffer today can be prevented, reversed, and often cured by lifestyle changes that nearly everyone can make at home.

And yes, you, along with Mother Time, can learn how to turn back that clock.

NOTE: As you read the chapters in this book, look for clues to the lifestyle factors that made such a difference in Hattie's health.

Part I

DISORDERS OF METABOLISM

The Worm and the Butterfly

Diets Don't Work

The worm writhed inside its cocoon. It had been there so long. The doors and windows had been sealed shut. There seemed no way out.

I was that worm. I could scarcely remember what it felt like to be free and in control of my life. For 30 years I had been increasingly hemmed in by external and internal habits. So many things had gone wrong. I thought as I struggled, *Why do I feel so trapped? Why can't I break out of this cocoon? Where is God? Am I to go to my death without realizing any meaning to my life?*

I'VE FINALLY LEARNED WHY DIETS DON'T WORK.

Somewhere in the dim past I had married and borne two wonderful children. But from the beginning the marriage was stressful. I didn't know how to cope, how to turn negative experiences into positive growth. When I felt down, I'd make my usual circle in the kitchen, beginning at the refrigerator, proceeding to the cupboard, moving to the freezer, then back to the refrigerator. As the years rolled on, so did the pounds. Then came the merry-go-round of dieting—10 pounds down, then 15 pounds back up. I couldn't keep it off. Year after year I struggled through the demoralizing routine of losing a little weight, then gaining back more. My self-esteem plummeted. "I want out! I want out!" I cried again and again, but I couldn't find a way. I had bound myself securely inside a cocoon of a bad lifestyle and depression. Though the thought terrified me, death seemed the only solution.

Finally my struggles ceased. I was worn out, tired of failure, tired of hating myself. In desperation I cried out, "Lord, if You don't do something for me I'm not going to make it!" Bitter tears flooded my cheeks as I gave up the fight.

Two weeks later I went to a summer revival meeting. I don't know why I ended up going, but I like to think the Lord gave me the necessary shove. One of the speakers, an epidemiologist and heart researcher from Loma Linda, California, quoted scientific data suggesting that most Western killer diseases, such as atherosclerosis, adult diabetes, high blood pressure, and heart disease, could be avoided—even reversed. The doctor talked about eating *more* and weighing *less*. He said that by markedly reducing the intake of fats, oils, sugars, cholesterol, and salt and by eating more wholesome grain products, beans, potatoes, fruits, and vegetables, we could lose unwanted pounds. He spoke with authority, showing us, step by step, how we could avoid the very things we dreaded.

I sought out the doctor and blurted out my story, one he'd probably heard a hundred times before. "Don't ever give up," he encouraged me. "The best is yet to come!"

God only knows how badly I wanted to believe that! A spark of hope appeared. Maybe I *could* become the woman I once had been. Maybe my marriage wasn't hopeless. As I returned to my room, my spark of hope burst into a blaze. My new lifestyle began with my very next meal. And the next morning I joined the exercise class.

There followed a year of intense and dramatic change for me, a metamorphosis from an old, over-weight, tired, listless "worm" into an energetic, slim-mer, healthier, happier "butterfly." It was a year that also brought me closer to God and to a new under-standing of how to incorporate His health principles into my daily life.

With new hope I began to dream again. With a new attitude I began to set goals. Most important, my attitude about God got straightened out. I realized He had been with me all the time, but was just waiting for me to give Him permission to work in my life. From this heart knowledge came the sweet return of my self-worth, and from that the healing of my marriage.

Physically I'm becoming younger, rather than older. My aches and pains have disappeared. Forty pounds have melted away, and I'm still losing. My blood pressure is down to 120/70, and my cholesterol is 139 mg/dl (3.6 mmol/l). I walk regularly and have as much energy and endurance as I had when I was 21.

As I emerged from my cocoon, people noticed the "new me" and began asking questions. What a splendid opportunity to share with them what I'd learned! I'm frequently called upon to do public speaking, telling my story to church and civic groups, and I do lots of counseling. I took a writing course at a local college and have become a published writer.

Now, on the fourth anniversary of my "cocoon breakout," I thank God again for all He has done for me. At times I have to pinch myself to believe that I'm the same woman who, only four years ago, was depressed, lonely, and suicidal. It is I—but with a whole new mind-set, new energy, and a drive to help others.

I've finally learned why diets don't work. Permanent weight control requires a total lifestyle change. I'm eager to share my experience with anyone who is tempted to feel too old, too tired, and too hopeless to go on fighting. Begin with your health. As that improves other good things will start coming.

Yes, Dr. Diehl, four years ago you wrote, "The best is yet to come." You were right! For me, the best did come. By putting into daily practice God's principles of healthful living, this worm became a butterfly.

NOTE: Grace stopped eating almost all refined and processed foods, choosing instead whole plant foods. (See pages 156, 157, "Eat for Health.") She also incorporated a daily exercise program, as well as other health-building life practices. (See pages 158, 159, "Live for Health.")

The Skeptical Reporter
Creeping Obesity

I have a nose for news, and to my journalistic instincts this sounded like something worth a story. After all, it isn't every day that a medical researcher from California comes to our small town in British Columbia.

The opening lecture of the series, "Live With All Your Heart," captivated not only the audience but this cynical newspaper reporter as well. When the day came for the health screening, I was among the 400 people who showed up. *Just out of curiosity,* I assured myself. I took the tests, and the results were not pretty.

"Years of double greaseburgers with cheese had taken their toll," I reported to my readership. My cholesterol level was 211 mg/dl [5.4 mmol/l] (a level below 160 is considered optimal), and my weight was just over 190—rather high for my 5'7" frame.

YEARS OF DOUBLE GREASEBURGERS WITH CHEESE HAD TAKEN THEIR TOLL.

"Dangerous," wrote the doctor at the bottom of my report.

It didn't take a genius to agree with him. The results floored me. I knew I was a little heavy, but I don't own a scale, and if someone had asked me to guess my weight, I'd have pegged it between 170 and 175. But 190? What a porker! I was so depressed I went out for a bacon-and-eggs breakfast to get me out of the poor mood the test results had put me in. I ate this breakfast slowly, because it was going to be the last one of its kind for a long time. That day would be a turning point for me.

The basic message of the health presentations was that North Americans are a bunch of gluttons who are killing themselves with the good life. Heart disease and cancer are taking a lot of lives, many of which could be saved with a better diet.

Hans Diehl's diet was easy enough to follow. He basically advocated common sense: "Eat the stuff that's good for you—fruits, vegetables, legumes, grains—unprocessed and unrefined."

∞

Several months later I published this follow-up report of my experience:

It took about a week for my desire for the doughnut and my craving for the burger to die. But getting used to snacking on bananas, oranges, and apples wasn't tough. The diet was easy to stick to because it allowed me to eat as much as I wanted of the right stuff and still lose weight. In the past six months I've eaten more per meal than ever before, but I still managed to bring my weight down to 150 by the time Hans Diehl returned for a six-month checkup on his health screen participants. And guess what? He didn't recognize me!

Every excess pound of fat shortens the life span by about one month.

"When I met you, even though you were young, you looked so devastated . . . so debauched." He paused. "And because I knew that newspaper people live on caffeine, cigarettes, and stress, I had little hope for you."

"Yes, and we tend to grab hamburgers on the way to a town council meeting and fries on the way home," I added.

The most surprising aspect of my success is that I didn't follow the diet religiously. Hans Diehl advocated total vegetarianism—not even chicken, fish, or dairy products, which also pack on the pounds and cholesterol points. I usually indulged in roast chicken or pizza once a week, mostly as a reward for doing so well during the other six days of the week, but partly because I still kind of missed them.

You can imagine how nice it is not to have 40 extra pounds to pack around, but the mental improvement is something I didn't expect. It begins when people start noticing you're losing weight. Few things are better for morale than people telling you you're looking good. Before you know it, you've traded in the baggy sweatshirt and ill-fitting jeans for dress pants, a shirt, jacket, and tie. Then people really start to notice a difference. Not only are they commenting on the weight loss; they're also impressed with the change in attire and the improved outlook and attitude.

Even so, the good doctor has his skeptics, most notably restaurant and butcher shop owners. He doesn't do much for their business. But as you can imagine, I am no longer skeptical of the health principles he taught, and my restaurateur friends with salad bars are still making a fair buck off me.

But seriously, I, along with many others in this town, owe a lot of thanks to the heart study team. They've made us look and feel a lot better—and probably added a few years to our lives.

Extra weight is bad news. Even as little as 10 extra pounds can increase mortality figures (shorten life). Overweight people are at higher risk for heart disease, high blood pressure, and many cancers. They are five times more likely to develop adult diabetes. They have more gallbladder disease, osteoarthritis, and back pain.

The good news is that the rewards of losing excess weight are enormous.

NOTE: See pages 156-159 ("Eat for Health" and "Live for Health") for Len Logan's basic lifestyle changes.

The Soda Pop Girl
Beverages

Ruby Lee was beautiful. She was also the best operating room nurse I've ever known. I was an anesthesiologist in those days, and we worked together over a span of 15 years. I first met Ruby when she was 21, about three months after she'd graduated from nursing school in Bangkok, Thailand. I was a new missionary doctor, who had recently joined the hospital staff. I was immediately attracted to this bright, friendly, energetic woman, and we became good friends.

> HER TRIM, PETITE FIGURE BROADENED AND THICKENED. HER FACE BEGAN TO PUFF.

I quickly learned a few things about tropical Thailand. Every day was humid. The seasons consisted of the hot season, the hotter season, and the rainy season. During the rains the humidity became even worse. Because the city water was unsafe to drink, we boiled our water, cooled it, and stored it in jars in the refrigerator. Away from home we drank soda.

In those early days there was no air-conditioning in the operating room. Later, when it was installed, the electricity would frequently go off for indefinite periods, and the machines themselves broke down fairly regularly. About midmorning of every operating day Ruby Lee brought in bottles of ice-cold soda. She would lift the face masks of the perspiring surgeons and nurses and hold the bottles as they gratefully gulped down the cool liquid through a straw. Every morning our operating room refrigerator was stocked with bottles of orange-flavored soda to which the operating room personnel had unlimited access. Those drinks became a survival tool.

During the next few years Ruby married and had children. Her trim, petite figure broadened and thickened. Her face became puffy. I often thought of the earlier days and felt saddened by what I saw happening to her body.

About that time I started a weight control class in one of the hospital classrooms. I was pleased that Ruby chose to join. As the weeks went by most of the class struggled hard to lose a pound here and there. Some became discouraged and quit. But Ruby was different. Week after week her weight went down, down, down. When asked for the secret of her success, she would give only a bemused smile. I watched with delight as the attractive, shapely woman I had once known emerged once more.

On the last day I asked various class members to share the particular part of the program that had been most helpful to them. As we worked our way around the circle, it was finally Ruby's turn. She again smiled her bemused smile, and I held my breath. But this time she was ready to talk.

"I actually made only two changes in my lifestyle," she said. "I joined a gym and exercised for one hour every day after work—and I stopped drinking soda. I've lost 40 pounds and am back to my nursing school weight. I feel better than I have for years."

Americans consume twice as much soda as they did 25 years ago—a habit that contributes to obesity, tooth decay, and loss of bone mass. In fact, research reveals that obesity rates have risen in tandem with soda consumption.

Soda pop is the number one source of refined sugar in the American diet. We now average 54 gallons of soda per year for every man, woman, and child in this country. (A 12-ounce can contains 10 to 12 teaspoons of sugar.) The problem is serious enough that the National Institutes of Health in Washington, D.C., are now recommending that people drink water instead of sugary soft drinks—sometimes referred to as liquid candy.

Water is the perfect beverage. It has no calories, requires no digestion, does not irritate, and is exactly what the body needs to carry on the life processes. How much should we drink? We should drink enough to keep the urine pale—at least six to eight glasses of water a day.

HOW MANY CALORIES DO YOU *DRINK* IN A DAY?		
Drink	**Amount**	**Calories**
Coffee, cream, and sugar . . . . 1 cup		75
Orange juice . . . . 1 cup		110
Soft drinks, juice, punch. . . . . 12 oz.		140
Diet soft drinks. . . . . 12 oz.		0
Nonfat milk . . . . 1 cup		90
Whole milk. . . . . 1 cup		160
Milk shake . . . . 12 oz.		425
Beer. . . . . 12 oz.		150
Cocktail 1		150
Mineral water. . . . . 12 oz.		0

The Price Is Too High

Failure Is Costly

I was what the doctors call "morbidly obese." What horrible words!

I felt OK, but my husband pressured me to sign into a live-in health center. After I started the program, I fell in love with the place. I was impressed with the lifestyle and began to take some positive steps. My husband came with me. I actually thought he needed the program more than I did, because he'd already had heart bypass surgery. But he's stubborn—wouldn't admit it. Anyway, I really stuck with the program for six months. I lost 40 pounds and began to feel a lot better.

> I WOULD COOK ALL THE GOOD FOOD FOR MY HUSBAND EVERY DAY, THEN I WOULD FILL UP ON JUNK.

Then I hit a snag and fell off the wagon. Once off, it's extremely hard to get back on. By this time my husband had become a firm believer in this lifestyle—and he was getting results. He'd lost weight, his cholesterol was now in the ideal range, and he exercised daily, either outdoors or on the treadmill.

And me? I would cook him all the good food every day, then I'd fill up on junk. It's hard to explain; it's embarrassing; it's totally irrational! But it's what happens to many of us, especially those of us who have a very long way to go.

Since I am fairly young, I seemed to be fine for

quite a while. But the body can take only so much abuse. My joints began to hurt. It was harder to walk, harder to do my work. My blood pressure crept up. A painful, gouty arthritis flared up. Diabetes showed its ugly head, followed by a painful stomach ulcer. I was living on medication. It wasn't worth it. It was too big a price to pay.

So now I'm back at the health center again. My husband didn't have to push me. I'm the aggressor this time, and I mean business. I want to live. I want my health. God wants me to have these things. I'm determined to take God with me into this restart. The really sad part is that all this suffering would have been totally unnecessary if I had just stuck to the principles I learned three years ago. What a price to pay for stubborn pride!

My Best Friends Were My Dogs
Life-threatening Obesity

I mean it! I'm 42 years old, and a few months ago I weighed 290 pounds. I avoided people because they either pitied me or preached at me. I guess I was pitiful—I could not walk even a half block without severe leg pain. My knees and feet hurt so badly that my physician wanted to put me on a disability pension. But I wasn't ready to give up on life yet. Actually I was raised a good Christian, but like so many of my peers, I paid little attention to my health. I ate what I pleased.

It took a lot of suffering to finally wake me up.

When I heard about Hans Diehl's "Eat More and Weigh Less" health lecture, I thought, *Just what I need.* The week before I had managed to go without dough-nuts for a whole week—then felt so deprived I ate a dozen at one sitting. Yes, I definitely needed help.

After that first lecture I kept going and attended the entire four-week Coronary Health Improvement Project (CHIP). I bought a book and some cassette tapes and followed the instructions carefully at home. It felt good to start caring for my body in God's way.

My closest friends were my dogs, because they did not insult me.

It's been six months now, and I'm sure you would notice a big difference. I have dropped 100 pounds. I plan to lose another 30 pounds slowly to reach my normal weight. I have to tell you, it's true what they say about eating a lot of high-fiber plant food! With these changes in my diet I haven't felt hungry at all.

I'm like a new person! My breathing is normal. I can see my feet. I walk six miles a day without pain. My migraines have disappeared. I work full-time. I'm back in church.

But Hans Diehl made one mistake. He said this way of eating would save money. Have I got news for you! The program cost me a lot: I had to buy all new clothes! I'm not complaining, though. No, I'm not complaining. Every way I look at it, I got a real bargain.

∽

So how did he do it? Arnold learned that excess weight happens when the calories in the food eaten exceed the calories used for physical activity and maintenance of body functions. The leftover calories are stored as fat. Arnold also learned that different kinds of food are handled in quite different ways by the body. Here are the basic principles of his dietary lifestyle change:

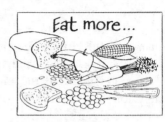

Eat more...

- Fresh and steamed vegetables, but go easy on sauces and salad dressings.
- Whole grains: cooked cereals, brown rice, whole-grain breads, pasta.
- Fresh whole fruits.

These *foods as grown* are filling, nutritious, high in fiber, inexpensive, and low in calories.

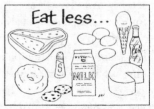

Eat less...

- Refined, processed, and concentrated foods. They are high in calories and price, and low in nutrients and fiber.
- Meat and rich dairy products. While these foods are nutritious, they have zero fiber and bulk, and are very high in fat, cholesterol, and calories. Meat and cheeses, for instance, carry 60 to 80 percent of their calories as fat.

Other basic health principles:

- *Drink six to eight glasses of water a day.* Save sodas and other caloried beverages for special occasions.
- *Walk briskly every day.* Keep at it until you can walk 60 minutes without fatigue or shortness of breath.
- *Beware of weak moments.* If one cookie leads to a dozen, don't eat the first one. Don't buy problem foods. If they are not around, you won't be tempted. If you feel bored, frustrated, or lonely, go for a walk, drink a glass of water, read a book, call a supportive friend. Or you can feast on natural foods such as semifrozen grapes, juicy melons, or crunchy carrot sticks.
- *Tie into spiritual resources.* God doesn't make nobodies. He created you for health and prosperity (see 3 John 2).

He Wanted to Go to Rio

Adult Type II Diabetes

Marvin really wanted to go to Rio de Janeiro. The president of his company and a number of delegates were going to Brazil to meet leaders from other countries. As head of security, his job was to arrange for their safety and protection and oversee the operation once they arrived. It was an exciting assignment, and also the chance of a lifetime to see one of the world's most beautiful cities.

But Marvin was having serious health

ONLY 49,
MARVIN
DEFINITELY WAS
NOT READY TO
BE TOSSED ON
THE SHELF.

27

problems. He was overweight, his blood pressure was too high, and even daily injections of 52 units of insulin were not controlling his diabetes. He'd had these problems for several years, but despite following everything his physicians told him to do, he kept getting worse. As the time neared for the trip he felt so sick and discouraged he knew there was little chance he could go.

His boss urged him to go to a live-in health center that specialized in problems such as his. At 49 Marvin was definitely not ready to be tossed on the shelf. After praying about it, he determined to go and fight for his life.

At the health center he faced a new diet, new concepts of health, and a new lifestyle. He'd been careful about sugar for years, but now he was taken off all refined and processed food, as well as all animal products. He learned how important an unrefined, high-fiber diet is for diabetics in that it helps stabilize blood sugar levels. He also learned how critical weight control is in the management of diabetes. Excess fat—on the body or in the diet—plays a pivotal role in adult-onset diabetes (Type II). It seems to deactivate the insulin, making it less effective in moving glucose (blood sugar) out of the bloodstream and into the cells, where it is needed as fuel. He found that the very low-fat, high-fiber diet allowed him to eat a higher volume of food with fewer than half the calories he was used to consuming. Even with his heavy exercise program of walking and hiking as many as 15 miles a day, he assured us that he never felt hungry at all. Additionally, exercise helped him lower his blood pressure, lose weight, reduce his insulin needs, banish depression, condition his body, and gave him a welcome sense of well-being.

At the end of the month his results were so amazing he told us he wouldn't have believed them if they hadn't happened to him. He had lost 22 pounds, and his blood pressure had normalized without medication.

"Praise the Lord! My blood sugar is staying within normal limits *without any insulin!* After 17 years I feel like a man out of prison—free at last. I can't remember ever feeling better in my life."

Six months later he sent us this report:

"I've now lost a total of 35 pounds, bringing me to my normal weight. I walk faithfully, seven miles a day, rain or shine. I joined a gym so that when the weather is bad I can work out there. My blood sugar and blood pressure remain normal, and I continue to feel like a young man. I wish I could tell the world about this lifestyle! And yes, I went to Rio."

Diabetes occurs when the body is unable to handle glucose (blood sugar) that builds up to dangerous levels in the blood. There are two kinds of diabetes, Type I and Type II.

Type I, Insulin Dependent Diabetes Mellitus (IDDM), commonly called juvenile diabetes, usually occurs in childhood or youth and can be hereditary. These diabetics cannot survive without insulin. About 5 to 10 percent of all diabetics are of this type.

Type II, Non-Insulin Dependent Diabetes Mellitus (NIDDM), is called adult-onset diabetes because it generally hits around midlife as people get older and fatter. These diabetics usually have plenty of insulin, but something blocks its action. About 90 percent of diabetics are Type II.

In the early stages there are few symptoms—perhaps some increase in urinary frequency, thirst, and an increased appetite. More than 16 million Americans are estimated to have the disease, but half don't know it yet. Complications appear later on. They include:

- eye problems (diabetes is the leading cause of new blindness);
- numbness in the feet and legs that can lead to amputations;
- kidney disease, which is 18 times more common in diabetics; and
- an acceleration of atherosclerosis, increasing the risk for heart attacks, making diabetes one of the leading causes of death in North America.

Simple lifestyle changes, such as Marvin made, produce near-miraculous results. A high-fiber, very low-fat diet apparently energizes and reactivates the body's natural insulin that can now move the glucose (blood sugar) into the cells where it belongs. As a result, elevated blood sugar levels often normalize within weeks, reducing and sometimes canceling the need for insulin injections. Daily active exercise is another effective way of helping the body use up its excess blood sugar. Most adult-onset diabetics are overweight, and normalizing weight will be a major factor in reversing their disease progression.

By utilizing these same principles, Type I diabetics will need less insulin and find their blood sugar levels easier to control. Good control, in turn, decreases the risk of complications.

A simple, inexpensive blood sugar test will help you know if you are at risk.

⌒

Sample Breakfast

1   cup oatmeal
½   cup soy or nonfat milk
1-2   slices 100 percent whole-wheat bread
1   banana (slice half over oatmeal; mash half for toast topping)
1   orange (peel and eat in sections)

Rx for Adult Diabetes

- Very low-fat diet (see "Reversal Diet," p. 153)
- High-fiber diet to stabilize blood sugars
- Active daily exercise to help body burn up excess blood sugar and fatty acids
- Most important: normalize weight. Often this is all that's necessary to reverse this disease. (See page 155 for your ideal weight.)

Diabetic at 17

Juvenile Type I Diabetes

Sandy was a typical American child, raised on a rather typical American diet of sodas, burgers, sweetened dry cereals, white bread, doughnuts, popcorn, candy bars, hot dogs, and french fries. She liked to practice the piano and make her own clothes, and she excelled at her studies. She never worried about her health, although she had several relatives who were quite obese and had something called "diabetes." Sandy didn't even know what that word meant.

I BECAME DEPRESSED AND BITTER, BLAMING GOD FOR GIVING ME THIS DISEASE.

During her last two years in high school, however, Sandy noticed that she could eat large amounts of food without gaining weight. "I just thought I was one of those fortunate people with a high metabolism," she says.

But by her seventeenth birthday Sandy had to face the fact that she had diabetes. "Although I was stunned initially," she says, "I know the Lord helped me accept my disease. I saw it as a challenge. I followed the prescribed American Diabetes Association [ADA] diet and began a vigorous aerobic exercise program. For a while I did well."

By the time she finished college Sandy's diabetes had edged out of control, and she was unable to go on to graduate school. "I was keenly disappointed and began to harbor self-pity and resentment toward this disease I couldn't seem to control. I became depressed and bitter and began blaming God for giving me this disease. I nursed my misery for about a year. Then one day during my devotional time I had a dramatic confrontation with the Lord. I began to see how self-centered and unproductive my life had become. I was now ready to turn to God for help."

Through several providential happenings, Sandy secured a job as a secretary for a well-known health center. She keenly observed the patients who came, especially the ones with diabetes. She noticed they were put on diets that were very low in fat and very high in fiber. It was quite different from the more traditional ADA diet. As she observed the results she became motivated to go beyond her lacto-ovo-vegetarian diet. She stopped using milk, eggs, and cheese. Then she began to eliminate most processed and refined foods and oils.

The results? Her daily insulin requirement decreased from 55 to 32 units per day. Sandy continued to exercise in earnest—walking, jogging, and cross-country skiing. Eventually she was able to stabilize her blood sugars with only one daily injection of insulin instead of two.

"Dealing with diabetes is not easy," she says, "especially when you are young. But God has taken away the bitterness and my frustration. He helps me live, day by day, without becoming overwhelmed by my problems. I can say now that I'm excited to see God working in my life, helping me grow physically, mentally, and spiritually as I learn to cooperate with Him and His health laws."

Sandy's diabetes is usually found in younger people. That's why it is called juvenile, or Type I, diabetes. However, more recently chilling reports have come in that obesity-related Type II diabetes, commonly considered a disease of middle age or later, is now turning up in children.

Many published studies have shown that 50 to 75 percent of Type II diabetics can be off drugs and needles within eight weeks by following the Reversal Diet (see page 153). Studies have also documented that many Type I diabetics will have much better blood sugar control with lowered insulin requirements on the same program. And since this dietary approach markedly lowers blood cholesterol levels, the serious vascular complications affecting the eyes, ears, kidneys, heart, and feet can be reduced greatly, if not prevented entirely.

The Nurse Should Know

Diabetic Neuropathy

This is really embarrassing. I am a 55-year-old registered nurse who has taught nursing for many years. I should have known better! Actually, I did. But I didn't take my problems seriously. I cooked things I liked with lots of butter, eggs, and cheese. I also continued eating plenty of pork and chicken and drank lots of beer. *I'll do better next week,* I kept telling myself.

I had plenty of warning. I'd been overweight for

several years. Then I developed hypertension that I tried to control with drugs. Next came diabetes, and for nearly 10 years I've treated it with oral insulin. After a while my feet and legs developed tingly and crawly sensations and began to turn numb. Then the pains started and kept getting worse.

Finally I had to take codeine in order to sleep at night. The bottoms of my feet felt as if they were on fire all the time. I had several episodes of gout [a very painful type of arthritis] that caused my big toe joint to become red and swollen, adding to my misery.

The day came when I could no longer walk, not even in my softest slippers and on the softest carpet. It felt as though I were stepping on razor blades. I finally got serious, and that's why I signed in for *I KEPT TELLING MYSELF, "I'LL DO BETTER NEXT WEEK."* treatment at this health center, hoping they could help me.

The staff members explained that once diabetes attacks the nerves of the legs and feet they rarely recover. This is a serious situation, because as the numbness increases, the risk of injury and infection also increases. Since diabetes progressively impairs the circulation, often an injury or infection will not heal, causing gangrene to set in, and amputation often follows.

I knew all this. I should have come sooner. But I begged them to do what they could. Perhaps the progression of the damage to the nerves could be stopped. I promised to do everything I could to cooperate.

Kate was as good as her word. She accepted and

adjusted well to our Reversal Diet (see page 153), a plant-based diet that's low in fat (10 percent of calories) and high in fiber. She ate no refined or processed foods and eliminated all animal products. She didn't complain about the food, and soon began to relish it.

During her first few days Kate could barely walk around the flagpole—about 200 feet. But her distance increased with time. She began to lose weight, and her blood pressure dropped so much that her medication had to be reduced and finally discontinued. She also learned how to keep her blood sugar within normal limits with only small doses of insulin.

The most amazing results, however, related to her diabetic neuropathy, which she'd had for nearly five years. Her legs and feet gradually began to recover sensation. Physicians at the health center were impressed, and Kate became Exhibit A for visiting doctors and other health professionals.

Kate was not shy about demonstrating her improvement. "I know it is very unusual for diabetic neuropathy to begin to reverse itself the way my feet have. It is a miracle for which I thank God."

NOTE: Dr. Milton Crane, a research scientist working with Weimar Institute in California, has treated a number of patients with diabetic neuropathy with encouraging results. He is following these people carefully to determine how long their improvement continues and how much it relates to the ability to control the disease once they get home.

Part II

The Turnaround

Heart Disease With Angina

Hank Delmont was a farmer. For years he worked with efficient farm machinery equipped with air-conditioned cabs. This considerably altered his once-active life. He eventually began to experience angina (heart pain). It finally got so bad he couldn't get out of bed and go to the bathroom without pain. When he finally went to the doctor and had an angiogram, he was told that his heart disease was so extensive that bypass or other surgical procedures were out of the question.

You mean this no-fat diet is cleaning out my blood?

"Hank," his doctor said, "medically there just isn't any more we can do for you. I'm sorry." Hank was given several medications, mostly to control the pain, and sent home to put his affairs in order.

But his daughter wasn't ready to give up. She heard about a live-in health center out West that might help, and she urged him to go. He wondered if the expense would be justified—after all, he was at the end of the medical rope. Then the pain became so severe he decided to go.

Kind, friendly people welcomed him, and after a thorough physical evaluation his physician met with

37

Hank and his wife to talk about his problems.

"Even though people are born with clean, flexible arteries that should stay that way throughout life, the arteries of most Westerners and people in developed countries are clogging up with cholesterol, fat, and calcium," the doctor explained. "This concoction gradually hardens and eventually chokes off needed oxygen supplies, a process known as atherosclerosis.

"During World War II most Europeans were forced to change their eating habits from their customary diet of meat, eggs, and dairy products to a more austere diet of potatoes, grains, beans, roots, and vegetables. The surprising result? A dramatic decrease in heart attacks, which lasted for several years."

"That makes sense to me," Hank commented. "I've been a farmer most of my life, and a typical breakfast for me has been three eggs with sausage and bacon, fried potatoes, and coffee. My other meals weren't a whole lot better. I guess"—Hank stopped to clear his throat—"I guess I just ate myself into this condition. I didn't know any better."

"You aren't alone," the doctor said gently. "Heart disease now strikes a deadly blow to four out of every 10 people in North America. Medical science has finally come to realize that diets high in fat and cholesterol produce elevated levels of blood cholesterol and heart disease. The good news is that diets *very low* in fat and cholesterol can markedly reduce blood cholesterol levels. This in turn reduces coronary risk and can facilitate plaque reversal."

"So maybe there is hope for me, if I change my diet?" Though his voice quavered, Hank's eyes brightened. "Is a wrong diet the main cause of heart disease?"

"The most serious risk factor by far is an elevated blood cholesterol, which reflects the diet. Fifty-year-old men with cholesterol levels more than 295 mg/dl (7.6 mmol/l) are nine times more likely to develop atherosclerosis than men the same age with levels under 200 mg/dl (5.1 mmol/l). A 20 percent decrease in a man's blood cholesterol level lowers his risk of a heart attack by about 50 percent."

There are other important risk factors for heart disease. For example:

• By age 60, smokers are 10 times more likely to die from heart disease than are nonsmokers. About 30 percent of all coronary deaths a year are related to smoking.

• In North America one in every three adults has high blood pressure. Such a person is three times more likely to die of heart disease and stroke than a person with normal blood pressure is.

• Obese men are five times more likely to die of heart disease by age 60 than men of normal weight. Other risk factors include diabetes, elevated triglycerides, sedentary lifestyle, and stress.

"All of the above risk factors can be controlled by changes in diet and lifestyle," Hank's doctor told him. "Heredity, age, and gender are also risk factors, but these we can't control. Fortunately, they are the least important."

Hank visibly relaxed. "So I *do* have a few things going for me. I don't smoke, I'm not overweight—and I don't have diabetes!"

His doctor smiled. "That's right. However, as you know, you *do* have a very advanced case of coronary heart disease. And yes, you *can* get better. Just be patient."

During the first week Hank could do little more than walk to the cafeteria and to physical therapy, but the chest pain was gradually lessening. By the end of the second week he could walk a half mile without pain. Hank was delighted, but curious. "Why am I getting better so soon?" he asked the doctors. "There hasn't been time for collateral circulation or plaque reversal to occur." (Hank had learned these terms from the medical lectures.)

"That's a good question," the doctors told him. "People don't realize that when they eat a high-fat diet, the excess fat thickens their blood, and circulation becomes sluggish. It is possible to observe this milky-looking blood in the small vessels of the human eye. Fat-thickened blood is sticky, causing red blood cells to adhere to each other in bunches. These clumped blood cells cannot carry their full load of oxygen and are unable to navigate tiny capillaries."

"You mean this no-fat diet I'm eating is cleaning out my blood?" Hank asked incredulously.

"You are actually eating a low-fat diet—in your case, very low, about 10 percent of your daily calories. Because this fat occurs naturally in your food, you don't see it."

"So you can actually slip more oxygen to my heart muscle by thinning out my blood!" Hank exclaimed.

"That's the idea. Every little bit of extra oxygen that reaches your heart helps it grow stronger and decreases the pain of angina."

"So it's possible for me to get better." Hank was trying to absorb the concept.

Hank continued to improve gradually. After four weeks he could walk two miles a day—slowly, but without pain. Because of his precarious situation, Hank decided to stay another month. His endurance continued to improve, and at the end of the second month he could walk a little more than four miles a day without angina pain. He didn't do this all at one time, but in bits and pieces throughout the day.

When Hank left for home he carried his own suitcases to the car. He reports that he can now work nearly all day. He goes slowly, sometimes taking as much as a week to accomplish what he could once do in a day. "But I'm doing it without pain, as long as I pace myself. I have a long way to go, but little by little my endurance is increasing. I feel my recovery is a direct blessing from God, and I thank Him daily. I'd like to share my experience with others who might feel that the way is too hard or that recovery is too slow. Stick with it. Life is worth it."

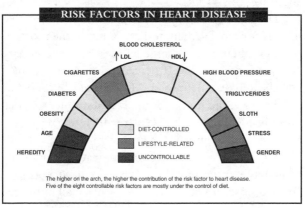

RISK FACTORS IN HEART DISEASE

BLOOD CHOLESTEROL
↑LDL   HDL↓

CIGARETTES   HIGH BLOOD PRESSURE
DIABETES   TRIGLYCERIDES
OBESITY   SLOTH
AGE   STRESS
HEREDITY   GENDER

DIET-CONTROLLED
LIFESTYLE-RELATED
UNCONTROLLABLE

The higher on the arch, the higher the contribution of the risk factor to heart disease. Five of the eight controllable risk factors are mostly under the control of diet.

41

Springing the Heart Trap
Silent Heart Disease

Feeling miserable from the flu, Donald Conway went to see his doctor. After a thorough examination the doctor delivered his verdict. "You've got a heart problem. We'd better schedule an angiogram right away."

Donald looked at the doctor in shocked disbelief. "I—I can't have a heart problem," he sputtered. "Why, I jog every day, play golf, climb mountains, fly planes. How could I have heart disease?"

"Many people don't realize that half of all fatal heart attacks occur without a single warning symptom," the doctor explained. "You are fortunate to discover your heart disease before it has seriously damaged your heart, while you can still do something about it."

Despite Donald's doubts, the angiogram revealed four major blockages in his heart arteries, the most serious one being in the large left descending coronary artery. It was nearly 80 percent obstructed. Donald felt cheated and depressed. He pictured himself fiddling around the house for the rest of his life, a dismal outlook for a man who went regularly on major safaris, collecting animals for various museums.

Explaining the angiogram, the cardiologist confirmed the diagnosis. "Yes, you do have coronary artery disease. If you want to be active at all in the future or to fly again, you should have bypass surgery. A clean vein is taken from your leg and sutured into the coronary artery tree so that the narrowed areas can be bypassed."

"Since my arteries clogged up, what about the veins?" Donald asked. "Will they clog up too?"

"Yes, they can. Around 15 to 30 percent of by-pass veins clog up within the first year after surgery. But if you make it through the first year, the bypasses are usually good for five to eight years."

"Is there any other choice?" Donald asked. "Seems like I've read something about heart disease being treated with diet and exercise."

The doctor hesitated. "Yes, there is another option, but it involves serious lifestyle changes."

The doctor explained that in 1989 Dr. Dean Ornish enrolled 48 coronary patients, many of whom were candidates for bypass surgery, into a special study. He randomly assigned the men to different groups. Both groups were asked to quit smoking and to walk daily. Additionally, the first group practiced stress management principles and followed a very low-fat vegetarian diet with less than 10 percent of total calories as fat and no cholesterol. The second group was given the American Heart Association's "prudent diet" for heart disease. This diet allows 30 percent of calories as fat and up to 300 milligrams of cholesterol a day.

At the end of the year Dr. Ornish reported that those on the very low-fat vegetarian diet not only had dropped their average blood cholesterol level by 40 percent but were actually enabling their narrow, plaque-filled arteries to widen, allowing more blood and oxygen to reach the heart muscle. The heart disease had, in fact, begun to reverse itself. The older men with the more advanced disease actually had the best results.

The group on the so-called prudent diet, however, had had virtually no cholesterol drop, and their coronary arteries showed progressive narrowing. Their heart disease had actually gotten worse.

"This is terrific news," Donald enthused. "Why don't more people know about this? And why did they introduce me to bypass surgery as my first option?"

"The Reversal Diet is a very low-fat vegetarian diet that contains no animal products except egg whites and nonfat milk. Sad to say, most people who are used to the rich Western diet cannot conceive of making the kind of changes necessary to achieve these kinds of results. Too threatening.

"The situation today is well summed up in Dr. Dean Ornish's book *Program for Reversing Heart Disease*.* He says we've gotten to a point in medicine where it is somehow considered radical, or an ordeal, to ask people to stop smoking, manage stress better, walk, and eat a healthful diet. And it is considered conservative to saw people open and bypass the arteries or to slip balloons inside the arteries and squish them or put them on powerful drugs for the rest of their lives. I think our medical priorities are a little topsy-turvy."

"That is truly amazing," Donald commented. "I *want* to do this program—reverse my heart disease, the way Dr. Ornish's patients did."

"It's a difficult road," the doctor warned. "You will have to stick with this program for years, probably for the rest of your life."

"I'll do anything to avoid heart surgery," Donald told him, "even if I have to live on grass."

Donald proved as good as his word. In time he and his wife began to enjoy the simple, natural food, much like the diet prescribed for Adam and Eve in the Bible, where fruit, vegetables, grains, and legumes take center stage. He also gradually increased his walking/jogging from his usual 20 miles per week to 40 miles or more.

Results were not slow in coming. At the end of one month Donald's cholesterol level had dropped from 222 mg/dl (5.7 mmol/l) to a much safer 141 mg/dl (3.6 mmol/l). After one year his stress treadmill test showed considerable increase in exercise tolerance, and it showed even more tolerance at the end of the second year.

Early in the third year Donald went back to serious hunting. A safari to Nepal (home of Mount Everest) took him to elevations of 15,000 feet with no problems. Later he climbed the Tibetan plateau in China, at 16,000 feet. He has continued his hunting trips in the high mountains ever since.

At the five-year mark Donald's cardiologist told him, "Your treadmill stress test is within normal limits. I'm certain you've experienced reversal, although I don't think you should undergo the risk and expense of another angiogram just to prove it.

"You've made a believer out of me," the doctor added. "I've decided to follow this lifestyle myself!"

---

*Dean Ornish, M.D., *Program for Reversing Heart Disease* (San Francisco: University of California, 1990), p. 78.

She Thought She Was Doomed
Hereditary Heart Disease

When her youngest brother dropped dead of a heart attack, Ruth Racker panicked. She totally panicked. Seven brothers and sisters had died, one after the other, of heart and vascular problems. Her husband had died also.

At age 68 she was the only one left, and she already had had two heart attacks. She knew she could die any minute. Her doctor gave her several medications and told her to take good care of herself. There wasn't much more he could do. She knew that heart disease was in her family gene pool, and she felt doomed. At the end of her rope, she pleaded with God for help.

A few days later she found an article about Dr. William Castelli, who was the director of the famous Framingham Heart Study for many years. Dr. Castelli, now in his 70s, is the first man among his kin to turn 50 without suffering a heart attack.

"I'm living proof that you can beat the odds of heart disease, even if it runs in your family," he says.

While Dr. Castelli was still in his 30s he began to notice that people who had high blood cholesterol levels had the most heart attacks. His own cholesterol was 270 mg/dl (7.0 mmol/l). "That's when the light came on," he says.

He started jogging every day and cut down on his

dietary fat, adding more plant-based foods. He brought his total cholesterol down to 170 mg/dl (4.3 mmol/l), his LDL cholesterol down to 90 (2.3), and his HDL (the good one) from 49 (1.3) to a healthier 63 (1.6). Dr. Castelli pointed out the most important risk factors of heart disease.

• High total cholesterol and LDL levels and low levels of HDL cholesterol are among the strongest predictors of heart disease.

• High blood pressure increases the risk of heart attacks and strokes by as much as five times.

• Smoking triples the risk of heart disease.

Dr. Castelli insists that a healthy lifestyle doesn't have to take the pleasure out of life. A person can significantly decrease the odds of having a heart attack by simply substituting low-fat foods in place of high-fat foods and by taking brisk walks several times a week.

Ruth felt greatly encouraged by this story. She found a physician who guided her into a strict program of diet, exercise, and stress control that would not only prevent further damage to her arteries but would begin to reverse the damage already present. An eager and grateful patient, Ruth followed instructions to the letter. Eighteen months later she sent us the following report:

"Today I am off all medication, have no more angina, and feel full of energy. I care for my home, paint, do volunteer work, go aerobic dancing three or four times a week, and teach a Bible class at my church. I don't plan to retire until I'm 90. There's too much I want to do! Do you doubt my story? I wouldn't believe it either, except that it really happened to me."

Fourteen Extra Years
After Bypass

Three months after his triple coronary bypass, Father Fergus McGuinness experienced the return of his symptoms—pain, fatigue, frustration. He went back to see his physician.

"The surgery helped you some, but that is as far as we can go. Continue your medicines and try to control your stress. A few drinks might help. Maybe you should see a psychiatrist."

Father McGuinness became deeply depressed. After his surgery he had joyfully thrown away the medications he'd been gobbling by the handful. Did he have to start that old routine again? Would he end up an alcoholic, trying to endure the situation? Perhaps he *did* need a psychiatrist. But before he had a nervous breakdown, he heard about rehabilitation classes for people with heart disease. He signed into the next class.

MY TRIPLE CORONARY BYPASS LASTED ONLY THREE MONTHS.

The physicians at the health center explained to him that the symptoms often return after bypass surgery unless the factors that caused the condition in the first place are changed, namely a high-fat, low-fiber diet, coupled with a stressful sedentary lifestyle.

Father McGuinness learned that switching to a low-fat vegetarian diet, coupled with walking for 30 to 60 minutes every day, was essential. It took con-

48

siderable discipline for him to discard lifelong patterns and adopt health-building habits, but he persevered. Within a month his cholesterol had dropped 102 points, and he'd lost 17 pounds (8 kilograms). He felt 10 years younger.

Father McGuinness followed the program faithfully throughout the years that followed. He told us recently that what he had learned has extended his life 14 years so far. He is 74 years old now, works full-time, and has no plans to retire.

NOTE: In recent years most physicians have been advising heart surgery patients to enroll in rehabilitation programs.

The Moment of Truth
Cholesterol

I guess I asked for it. I'd been feeling a little stressed out, and I thought it was time for a checkup.

"Are you going to be all right?" asked the nurse, a little too solicitously for my liking, as she strapped my arm and drew near with the needle. "I mean, you're not going to faint, are you?"

I ONLY REGRET I DIDN'T START THIS LIFESTYLE SOONER.

No, I wasn't going to faint. Not from the pain, anyway. But the anticipation of a bad result always makes me less than an ideal patient. Nobody fainted at my blood-taking. It was all very undramatic, and they promised to call me when the results were in. Actually, I called them—several times—trying to find out the state of my body. I wasn't prepared for the call I received a few days later.

"Your cholesterol of 258 mg/dl (6.6 mmol/l) is very high," said the nurse. "The doctor wants you to begin medication immediately to get it down to more ideal levels of 150 to 170 (3.8 to 4.4 mmol/l)."

I walked to the pharmacy to pick up my medicine. Exercise is necessary to keep cholesterol moving, right? Well, wrong reasoning, actually, but a good start. And I started taking those little pills every day, without fail.

The moment of truth came after my return from the doctor's office, where I'd picked up a pharmaceutical company giveaway. On the back of the pamphlet I found a food chart that listed cholesterol and fat contents for a wide range of basic foodstuffs and prepared meals. It wasn't the first time I had seen such a chart, but this time I looked at it more closely. That's when something struck me with the force of a revelation. Clearly some foods are higher in cholesterol and fat than others. But the bottom-line reality is that fruits, grains, and vegetables have no cholesterol, are very low in fat, and high in certain fibers that help lower the blood cholesterol.

It's amazing how fixated we consumers have become on foods low in fat and cholesterol. We have all become inveterate food label readers. All the while the answer is staring us in the face. Back to basics! It's not a bad idea, especially dietwise.

Thousands of years ago the ideal diet was spelled out by our Creator. The Bible says God told Adam and Eve,

"I have given you every plant yielding seed which is upon the face of all the earth, and every tree with seed in its fruit; you shall have them for food" (Gen. 1:29, RSV).

It's been only four weeks since that moment of truth. Yesterday I had another blood test. The result was terrific! My cholesterol was down to 124 mg/dl (3.2 mmol/l)! My doctor took me off the cholesterol-lowering drug, saying, "You don't need this anymore. Your diet change certainly made a difference. Stay with it, and you won't have to worry about drug side effects, seeing the pharmacist, or seeing me!" Great news!

More good news is that I've lost weight, gained energy, regained an incredible taste appreciation for simpler foods and, very important, I'm feeling much better. What a way to be!

NOTE: We called Lincoln a year later to see how he was doing. "I'm doing fine," he reported. "My weight is down to what it was when I got married, which means I'm 30 pounds lighter. I only regret I didn't start this lifestyle sooner. I feel years younger."

The Midnight Call
High Risk

After pushing the "play" button on my phone answering machine in my apartment in Kalamazoo, Michigan, that night, I heard a fearful, begging voice: "When you have my HeartScreen results done, would you please call me tonight?"

Should I really return Bill Schley's phone call? It was nearly midnight. I had just finished evaluating the second set of the tests that had been taken by more than 500 people. These folks had enrolled in the four-week, 40-hour, educationally intensive Coronary Health Improvement Project (CHIP). The first set of HeartScreens had been taken and evaluated before the four-week intervention program began. Our program stresses a simpler lifestyle, daily walking, and an unrefined, plant-based diet that's very low in fat, sugar, and salt, but high in foods as grown.

NOW I AM HEALTHY BY CHOICE, NOT BY CHANCE.

Should I really call so late? After all, the clinical results about cholesterol, blood sugar, blood pressure, etc., would be made available tomorrow, on graduation day. Torn between reservations about calling so late and the urgency expressed in the message, I decided to call. Bill answered on the first ring.

"Please tell me about my blood cholesterol level," he asked with obvious anxiety. "Before I started CHIP it was 365 [mg/dl], and my triglycerides were 1,260 [mg/dl]. Have they improved?"

"Yes, indeed!" I answered. "Your cholesterol is now at 144 [mg/dl], and your triglycerides [the blood fats] are 251 [mg/dl]. You have reason to feel very good about what you have accomplished."

It was as if the line had gone dead. All was silent. Finally some sniffles, a sob, and then a quiet, somber voice said, "Dr. Diehl, you will never know what this means to me! Three months ago, when I applied for a major bank loan to expand my business, I was told the loan had been approved. The only thing needed to clinch the deal was an updated life insurance policy. I wasn't concerned when the insurance company sent a nurse to my home to draw some blood and to ask me some questions. After all, I was only 49, and I felt fine. The results, however, were disastrous. I was informed that my coronary risk was too high, and that I must either get my cholesterol and triglyceride levels way, way down or apply to another insurance company. It was suddenly clear—no insurance policy, no bank loan, and no business expansion. And my life was in danger to boot!"

It was under those circumstances that Bill Schley heard about CHIP. Needless to say, his motivation was strong, and he and his wife invested themselves with earnestness in the program.

Bill continued, his voice stronger, and I sensed his joy. "You can understand what this means to me, my family, my business, and my life! I am determined to maintain these results."

Five months later I received another phone call. It was no longer the hesitant, fearful voice that had answered my previous call. Now it was the voice of a self-confident business owner.

He had received his bank loan.

He had regained his health.

He was now optimistic about his future.

"I'm so glad that I learned how to take charge of my health," Bill continued. "So thankful for what CHIP taught me. Now I am healthy by choice, not by chance."

The Living Museum

Multiple Diseases

Imagine a museum full of different diseases. That was Connie. She had coronary heart disease, gout, hypertension, diabetes, and depression. On top of all that, she was overweight and constipated.

Finally Connie's physicians at the Ottawa Heart Institute told her there was nothing they could do for her that hadn't already been done. She had received a triple coronary bypass and, four years later, an angioplasty. In addition, she was taking 27 pills a day for her coronary heart disease, gout, hypertension, and depression, plus 60 units of insulin for her diabetes. She couldn't walk more than 100 yards without popping nitro pills. To add insult to injury, her cardiologist forbade her to fly, which quickly canceled her plans to spend the winter in sunny Florida.

CONNIE COULDN'T WALK 100 YARDS WITHOUT POPPING NITRO PILLS.

By now Connie was totally depressed and suicidal. Feeling like such a drag on her family, she asked her husband to put her into a nursing home. Instead he enrolled her in Ottawa's Coronary Health Improvement Project (CHIP). By this time Connie was ready to grasp at any straw of hope. She faithfully attended the entire 40-hour seminar. With her husband's help, she began living the lifestyle she had learned.

The result? Within six months she dropped 46

pounds and was down to three pills a day, with her insulin dose at half the previous level. She now walked three miles daily and swam on a regular basis. Instead of being depressed, she went on a health cruise to Alaska. Most of her pain was gone. Instead of $490 a month for medications, her bill was now $80.

Ten years later, and now 65 years of age, Connie is still healthy and strong. She and her husband love to travel. Last Christmas they sent a postcard from Perth, Australia:

"We are just now leaving for Hong Kong—and we are *not* traveling by boat! I thank God for leading me to CHIP and a whole new life. We are now living our golden years in a way we could only dream about before."

I Blacked Out

High Blood Pressure

I was at home, relaxing with the evening paper. As I got up to go to the bedroom, I blacked out. Two hours later my family found me still crumpled on the floor. They summoned the medics. My blood pressure was 210/160. I regained consciousness on the way to the hospital.

MY FAMILY FOUND ME CRUMPLED ON THE FLOOR.

At the emergency room my blood pressure was somewhat better, and they found no signs of a stroke or other catastrophe. I was given several medications and told, "Go home and take it easy for a few days—and lose some weight."

I went home and rested for a few days. I didn't know what to do with myself. I felt bored and ate even more than usual. I realized I wasn't getting better. In fact, I felt so lousy that it scared me into coming to this health center.

In college I was slender, athletic, and in top health. Even after going into the business world I took special precautions with my health. Until five years ago I worked out regularly at the YMCA. Even though my weight was creeping upward, I remained solidly muscular.

About that time events piled up on me. My wife became critically ill, needing round-the-clock care. My work included increasing amounts of travel. My business success involved me in more and more entertaining. Some days I not only had business dinners but business lunches and even business breakfasts. I knew I was eating too much rich food and exercising too little. But I saw no way out. Besides, I was feeling OK.

Then two years ago a painful attack of gout sent me to the doctor. He warned me that I would soon have serious health problems if I didn't lose weight and find a way to reduce the stress in my life. My blood pressure was already on the way up, and I was given medication to control it.

I realize now this experience was a wake-up call. It should have scared me into making some serious changes in my life. But at the time I had many pressing matters to attend to. Besides my wife's illness, I had important business appointments waiting and several trips lined up. I just couldn't get out of these obligations.

I am a chemical engineer specializing in the designing of chemical process plants for handling plastics. I travel all over the country—and much of the world—demonstrating and selling these processes and techniques. It's taken many years to build this successful business, and I wasn't about to let it fall apart. I took off a few days, lost a few pounds, and plunged back into my nonstop life.

A few months ago I began feeling increasingly fatigued. My efficiency at work fell markedly. My head seemed full of cobwebs. As my work deteriorated, cold fear edged into my consciousness. I blamed my problems on my medications and stopped taking them. Two months later—I blacked out.

"I'm sure that if I can just lose 40 pounds I'll be OK," I told the doctors at the health center. "I've heard that just getting the weight down is often all that is needed to return a high blood pressure to normal range."

∽

But Stephan wasn't going to lose 40 pounds while he was at the center. Even if he did, he'd probably put them right back on when he got home.

"While you are here, we want to help you develop a different lifestyle, one that will help you lose weight and keep it off, and that will normalize your blood pressure in more natural ways," we told him. "By combining regular, active exercise with a low-fat, high-fiber diet and hydrotherapy [hot and cold water treatments], we can help you improve the circulation of your blood. In addition, a low salt intake helps pull out retained fluid."

Excess weight in middle age also raises the risk of diabetes and coronary heart disease. Stephan's tests revealed that he had these problems as well. Away from the pressures and strains of work, Stephan relaxed and began enjoying his new lifestyle. By the second week he felt like his old self again.

Before he left, Stephan came to my office again, and I reminded him that he had not reached the one goal he came for. "No," he laughed. "I didn't lose 40 pounds; that was unrealistic. But I did lose 15 pounds, and I've learned how to work off the rest of my weight without starving. And so many other good things have happened. My fasting blood sugar is normal now. My blood pressure is down where it should be, even though the doctor cut my pills in half. My cholesterol has dropped to safe levels, and I have been walking six to eight miles a day without needing those nitroglycerin pills for my heart.

"But better yet, I've had time to reevaluate my life and obtain new perspectives. I realize that this is the kind of lifestyle God intended for us—not only to heal us, but to prevent these kinds of diseases in the first place. A few nights ago I totally rededicated my life to the Lord. I'm beginning to understand what is truly important in my life."

∞

Fourteen years later, when he was 76 years old, I met Stephan again. I hardly recognized him.

"No wonder," he said. "I've lost 70 pounds since

I saw you last. I am healthy and feel great. I feel as though I'm 40 years old again—the way I felt before all my problems started."

A PERSON WITH HIGH BLOOD PRESSURE IS

- three times more likely to have a heart attack
- five times more likely to develop heart failure
- eight times more likely to suffer a stroke than persons with normal blood pressure.

Hypertension is called the "silent" disease because there are no warning symptoms until a stroke or heart attack strikes. Be sure you have your blood pressure checked periodically, especially if you are over 50!

From Zombie to Fireball

Side Effects of Medication

I have hypertension," Frank told us, "and I'm taking medication that controls it. But I feel like a zombie. I just kind of wander around through my days, trying to do little things but accomplishing next to nothing. For a man who has lived a full and exciting life, the frustration is unbearable."

During his active life, this Christian pastor had pioneered much of the early mission work in remote areas of Central and South America.

"Even after retirement," he continued, "interesting challenges kept me involved. But then my weight crept upward, and so did my blood pressure. My worried doctor ordered medicines to control my blood pressure, hoping to prevent a stroke. However, the medicines put me in this unreal daze. I'd like to know if there is a better solution to this problem."

"There are two ways you can go," I explained. "The best way is to make significant changes in your lifestyle. For example, most high blood pressure responds rapidly to lifestyle measures, because a low-fat diet and regular active exercise work together to improve circulation of the blood. Also, the majority of hypertensives are sensitive to salt and receive considerable benefit from restricting salt intake, because it helps the body pull out retained fluid."

I WAS LIVING IN A ZOMBIE NETHERWORLD.

"Weight loss is very important as well," I continued, "because most blood pressures respond quickly to the loss of even a few pounds. Often normalizing weight is all that is needed to return a blood pressure to normal range."

Frank's other option was to try a different medication. Today there are many kinds of medications for hypertension available that control blood pressure without the need for weight loss, exercise, and salt restriction. His doctor could help him find one with fewer side effects.

"But you should know that medications do not *cure* high blood pressure, they only *control* it.

Medications are expensive and often need to be taken for life. And as yet no medication has been found that is totally free of side effects."

After thinking it over, Pastor Richards chose the first option—a simplified low-fat, low-salt diet, along with daily active exercise. He walked from three to five miles a day. He discovered that by eating high-fiber, whole-plant foods he could lose weight without feeling hungry. The pastor also stayed in touch with his doctor, who gradually lowered his medication as his blood pressure came down. One year later Pastor Richards gave us this report:

"It's still hard to believe what has happened to me. I'm 40 pounds lighter, and my blood pressure is normal without medication. I feel as though I've been re-born. I thank God for leading me to the right answers and for helping me out of a zombie netherworld into a vigorous reality full of exciting challenges."

SOME SALTY FACTS

- Americans and most other Westernized people eat 10 to 20 times more salt than the body needs.
- Excess sodium causes body tissues to hold extra water. This can result in weight gain and increased blood pressure.
- Every third American adult now has elevated blood pressure. For those over 65, the figure rises to 70 percent.
- Ideally we should use no more than five grams of salt a day, which is about one teaspoon.

FOOD PROCESSING—HIDDEN SALT

FOOD Natural State	SALT (mg)	FOOD Commercial, Processed	SALT (mg)
Apple (1 fresh)	5	Apple Pie (1 slice)	500
White Beans (1 cup)	12	Chili & Beans (1 cup)	3,000
Rice, Brown (1 cup)	12	Minute Rice (1 cup)	1,000
Wheat Flakes (2 oz.)	20	Wheaties (2 oz.)	1,850
Potato (1 fresh, 5 oz.)	20	Potato Chips (5-oz. bag)	3,500
Tomato (1 fresh)	35	Tomato Sauce (½ cup)	1,950
		Tomato Soup (1 cup)	2,200
Beef, lean	140	Corned Beef	2,360
Milk (1 cup)	300	Cheese, Amer. (2 slices)	2,050
Chicken (8 oz.)	300	Kentucky Fried Chicken (3-piece dinner)	5,600

Part III

The Couch Potato Fights Back
Traumatic Arthritis

Something was wrong. I felt it the moment I stepped into the office. I offered my cheeriest smile, but the woman's eyes were cold and belligerent. Her husband was carefully studying the carpet. I seated myself and picked up her chart, hoping for a clue to her hostility.

Back pain. Thirteen years.

My head started to ache. Chronic back pain—one of the most difficult and discouraging problems physicians face. I took a deep breath and looked up, my eyes meeting hers. I smiled again and spoke as gently as I could. "I want to help you. Where would you like to begin?"

She had been pushed too far; the dam broke. "I don't want to be here!" She spit the words out bitterly. "I've been forced to come. My own family did this to me, and I'm angry—furious!" Her eyes burned like hot coals. "I'm a mature adult, and I'm being treated like a 5-year-old child." Her voice, tight with emotion, wilted into a sob.

I jumped up. "I'm sorry," I heard myself saying. "There must be some mistake. We don't keep people

> LORINE WAS A CHRONIC CASE. SHE HAD WORN OUT HER DOCTORS, AS WELL AS HER LOVED ONES.

63

here against their will. Come, I'll help you arrange to go home."

She obviously hadn't expected this. She glanced at her husband. He shifted uncomfortably and continued to stare at the floor, stricken. Finally he looked up. "I—we—we did it because we want to help her," he said. "We didn't know she'd be so upset."

Lorine leaned back in her chair, her anger subsiding. She changed tactics. "Doctor, it would just be a waste of your time." Her voice was matter-of-fact now. "I've seen 11 doctors and had at least 100 X-rays. They say surgery won't help, and I've tried everything else."

EVERY EXCESS POUND INCREASES THE RISK OF CHRONIC BACK PAIN.

I sensed despair behind her words. She was a chronic case. She had worn out her doctors as well as her loved ones. She must insulate herself from further disappointment. I took her hands in mine. "Lorine, I *know* you can get better. You don't want to go on like this! Look, you're already here, and your care is paid for. How about giving our program a chance?"

Thank God, the words were right. The idea appealed to her. Lorine was basically a fighter, and she had been handed a ray of hope. Her gaze became distant as she weighed the idea. "Why not?" she said finally. "I'm a sinking ship anyway."

Lorine poured out her story. "I was once a vibrant, energetic woman, deeply in love with life. Besides being a wife to my minister-husband and mother to five children, I had my own business and was actively involved with my church.

"Thirteen years ago I fell down a stairway and injured my back. I was bedfast for some time, and my recovery was slow and incomplete. The past 13 years have been a blur of struggle and pain—always pain. I've had dozens of X-rays, but the answer is always the same: 'There is no operation that will help your problem.' My active life disintegrated, and I spent more and more time in bed or on the couch.

"Five years ago a severe knee injury made matters worse. My life became a round of sleeping, watching television, eating, and getting fat. I became a world-class couch potato," she concluded with a little laugh.

She was spunkier than I had thought. I explained that hers was a traumatic arthritis [an arthritis resulting from an injury]. In order for her back and knee joints to heal, they needed a better blood supply. I outlined her program:

- Diet. A low-fat, high-fiber diet removes the excess fat from the blood. (Excess fat slows down circulation by making the blood thicker and the blood cells sticky.)
- Exercise. Exercise stimulates collateral circulation, as well as helping the bones to preserve their minerals.
- Treatments. Hot and cold water treatments improve local circulation.
- Weight loss. Just as bridges have load limits, so do joints.

Having made up her mind, Lorine began focusing on the task at hand. She attended everything. She asked questions and borrowed books. Instead of getting more X-rays, Lorine went outdoors to walk. Actually, "walk" is an exaggeration. She waddled, slowly and painfully. She was carrying 65 excess pounds on her five-foot-one-inch frame. At first she could go only around the flagpole, grasping her husband's arm. But she did it, again and again. By the end of the month she was covering three to four miles a day.

There were no miracle drugs for Lorine, only an occasional pain reliever to dull her back pain. Food became her medicine. She ate three regular meals a day, with nothing between except generous drinks of water. Her diet consisted of a variety of plant foods—plenty of fruit and vegetables, beans and lentils, lots of grains, and a few nuts. Because she ate *foods as grown,* unprocessed and unrefined, she could eat a larger volume of food and still lose weight. Her diet was balanced so that she didn't feel hungry.

The following week Lorine literally bounced into my office. "This program really works! I feel good already. In fact, I haven't been this energetic in years." She paused, serious now, searching for the right words. "You know, this program isn't really that hard. Everything I'm doing here, I could do at home."

At the end of her time at the health center, Lorine was ecstatic. "I've lost nine and a half pounds, and my blood pressure is down from 170/114 to 130/80. My blood cholesterol has dropped from 266 mg/dl (6.8 mmol/l) to a much safer 194 mg/dl (4.9 mmol/l). And a threatening diabetic condition has disappeared."

Lorine did indeed "take the program home." A year later she dropped by—in a size 10 dress and with flowers in her hair. We could hardly recognize her. She was absolutely beautiful!

This is what she told us: "When I got home I

walked one hour every day and lived exactly as I lived here. Within a year I had lost 60 pounds. My back pain completely disappeared, as did my knee pain. I resumed caring for my home and family. I'm so glad I started fighting the right battles. Peter and I are still faithful to what we have learned, and I thank God for opening my eyes to ways in which I could cooperate in bringing about my own healing."

Sixty Pills and a Wheelchair

Rheumatoid Arthritis

Mary Ross was a legend at our health center. When I finally met her, she told me her story:

It's true. I was taking 60 pills a day and needed a wheelchair when I came to this health center. I couldn't raise my arms. I couldn't comb my hair. I couldn't climb stairs. I was nearly bedridden with advanced rheumatoid arthritis. Besides that, I had hypoglycemia. I carried snacks everywhere, even to church, to ward off the shakes and the disorientation that would follow. I was also overweight. A recent stroke blurred my vision, caused me to stagger, and made me feel dizzy and nauseated. When I walked, the landscape around me seemed to whirl, and I felt as if the pavement was coming up to hit me in the face. I lived in fear and dread of the next stroke, the big one. I was only 56 years of age.

In the 18 months prior to coming here I was very ill and spent thousands of dollars seeking medical help. I saw eight doctors, collected 60 pills (counting drugs and supplements), and took injections. But all the treatments and medicines did was take the edge off the pain.

I was finally advised to start cortisone, but I really feared that medicine. Rheumatoid arthritis is a long-term disease, and I did not want to become addicted. I improved a lot during my stay at the health center. I determined to stick to the new lifestyle I had learned when I got home.

It's hard to believe what's happened in the past three years! The hypoglycemia is gone, and I've lost 25 pounds. I now weigh 120 pounds, ideal for my height. I walk three miles a day with minimal pain and only an occasional mild flare-up of my arthritis. There is no observable residual from my stroke, and I've not had any more strokes. I've taken no pills for three years. In fact, I started to feel better the day after I stopped all those pills.

My husband, Tom, and I are very active socially and have lots of company. I cook them big, wonderful gourmet meals so they won't feel deprived because of me. But I hardly even taste the food. I have my potato, fresh vegetables, and a big salad. If I am ever tempted to cheat, I just stop and remind myself of the shape I used to be in. No, I haven't cheated. I've stuck with the diet and exercise program faithfully. We travel a lot, and I pack beautiful lunches, full of fresh, wholesome food. When we eat out, I have no trouble getting a baked potato and a fresh salad. I usually bring whole-wheat bread along.

Yes, I am strict. People cheat only themselves when they don't keep up their good health habits. Most people want a three-week miracle at the health center; they don't want to use their willpower. My only real problem is my mother. She continually offers me things I can't eat. She feels threatened when I refuse them. I guess she will never understand.

I wrote to Mary Ross recently, wondering if she was still OK. It had been 17 years.

"Yes, yes, yes!" she wrote back. "I'm still around, still healthy, and still faithful to my new lifestyle. I'm 73 now, busy, active, and feeling fine. I believe with all my heart that if it hadn't been for the new lifestyle that I learned, I wouldn't be around today."

❦

"Arthritis" is a general term for diseases of the joints. There are many kinds of arthritis, but rheumatoid arthritis is in a class by itself, in contrast to the more common osteoarthritis, which is usually related to injury or to wear and tear. Rheumatoid arthritis is thought to be one of the autoimmune diseases, many of which have an allergic component.

Rheumatoid arthritis results from inflammation of the joints, with redness, swelling, pain, and fever. Acute attacks tend to recur over the years, producing nodules and gradually stiffening and disfiguring the joints, most notably the wrist and finger joints.

Because rheumatoid arthritis is a chronic disease and joints heal slowly, short-term improvement is rarely dramatic. As time goes by, however, many of the people who chose to adopt a simpler diet and lifestyle have experienced long remissions.

In our experience the ones who have had the most effective results are those who, like Mary Ross, have been willing to adopt a very strict vegetarian diet that omits all animal products. This is not so surprising, since milk is the most common cause of food allergies, and eggs and beef are right up there as well.

The Crooked Back

Osteoarthritis

Y ou want to *what?*"

"I'd like to bicycle over the Rocky Mountains," Bob repeated. His voice was calm, even casual. "I have this doctor's appointment in Calgary on Friday. It's only 300 miles. If I start out Monday morning, I'm sure I can make it."

Theresa did a double take on this unbelievable husband of hers. Two years before, he had quit his job because of a painful, arthritic back. When it got worse, he had to give up doing even small jobs in his home workshop. He was so short of breath that he began driving his 22-year-old jalopy to the mailbox 50 yards away. Friends tried to comfort him. "You've worked hard all your life," they said. "You deserve a soft sofa and a *TV Guide*. You're finally free from the daily grind."

But freedom was no prize when it was coupled with constant pain. The soft sofa became a prison. Food, TV, cigarettes, and alcohol made up Bob's life, but none of them brought any pleasure. He tried to be cheerful. But he hit bottom the day he helplessly watched others cut, split, and stack his winter firewood. "I haven't one shred of ego left," Bob said. "I really don't think I'll live much longer. I'm already past the age when my father and brother died."

"You're only 66," his wife chided. But she couldn't lift his depression.

A few days later Theresa picked up a flyer in her doctor's office about a health seminar that was coming to town. The doctor noted her interest and urged her to go. "And be sure to take Bob along. Tell him it's doctor's orders."

Bob didn't need any urging. "Things can't get any worse," he said. They both signed up for the "Live With All Your Heart" seminar and began attending the meetings. The results of their health screen evaluations were a severe jolt. Bob knew he had arthritis, but he didn't know that he also had high blood pressure, high cholesterol, and diabetes. Theresa's results were no better. Additionally, both were overweight enough to be diagnosed as obese.

The message was simple: their diets were killing them. "Meat, dairy products, sugar, alcohol, salt, and tobacco—all the so-called good things of life—had to be removed from our home, or we would eat and drink ourselves into early graves," Theresa says now. Bob and Theresa also learned that rich food and sedentary living contributed to coronary heart disease, stroke, diabetes, hypertension, and osteoarthritis. But along with the bad news came the good news: these conditions could be improved, and often reversed, by healthful lifestyle changes.

Hope. That was what the Andersons needed. They willingly, even eagerly, decided to make the recommended changes. In one day meat, eggs, salt, alcohol, junk food, and caffeine disappeared from their house and their lives. Cold turkey. Bob's 35-year-old cigarette habit that he'd tried to break many times ended that night also.

The next day Bob slowly and painfully made his way to the mailbox. The effort exhausted him, but he did not give up. He even joked about it. "I must have been a sight," he said. "I was listing 45 degrees to port. I couldn't stand up straight."

They both began walking every day. One block; then two, three, five . . . They were on their way. By the fourth month the couple was ready to tackle hills and climb mountains. By the sixth month Bob's back pain had disappeared. "They say God can make crooked things straight," he deadpanned. "You can see He did it for me" (see Isaiah 40:4). He now stood straight and walked without a limp.

A few months later Bob bought a new 18-speed bicycle and gradually worked up to cycling 25 to 40 miles a day, six days a week. Within a year he had lost 32 excess pounds. His blood pressure, cholesterol, and blood sugar had normalized. He chopped his own wood and spent many happy hours in his workshop doing custom carpenter jobs.

So Theresa wasn't that surprised when Bob announced that he wanted to ride his bicycle to Calgary. The challenge of biking 300 miles over the Rocky Mountains excited him. Theresa packed the car with supplies and camping gear, and off they went. Three and a half days and 301 miles later, he had crossed the Rocky Mountains and arrived in Calgary.

"What? You came here on a bicycle?" his doctor asked in amazement. "I'm calling the paper."

In a few minutes reporters surrounded them, taking pictures and peppering them with questions. "We were always led to believe that martinis and rich foods were the rewards of a life of hard work," Bob told the reporters. "I used to have three eggs and six slices of bacon for breakfast. I would smoke three packs of cigarettes a day and have a couple drinks before dinner. At bedtime I'd have a large bowl of peppermint ice cream, topped with a gooey topping. We considered our health problems to be an inevitable part of aging. We wanted to enjoy all the good things we could get, but we felt miserable and weren't having any fun. In fact, at times we wished we could hurry up and die."

"But no more!" Theresa picked up the story. "We are no longer simply enduring retirement. We are living our lives to the hilt! We both have bicycles, and we love life on the road."

As their physical health improved, the couple grew spiritually. "We've been born again," they tell people. "Now we have a purpose, a sense of direction in our lives."

"I've decided that second childhood certainly beats the first," Bob observes dryly, "because there's no one around to tell you what you can't do."

A year later Bob bicycled 3,000 miles (4,800 kilometers) across Canada in 60 days to promote health—from Creston, British Columbia, to Ottawa, Canada's capital. As Bob bicycled through various cities, reporters would ask him what he thought made the difference in his health. He cited four CHIP principles:

1. Eat a simple diet of *foods as grown*.

2. Burn holes into the soles of your shoes, not the tires of your car.

3. Avoid harmful substances, such as tobacco, alcohol, caffeine, and other drugs.

4. Develop an attitude of gratitude. God didn't waste time making nobodies.

Bob Anderson, now in his 80s, is still active, still excited about life.

Just as a heart will weaken and ultimately fail when its arteries plug up with plaque, so joints begin to fail when the arteries supplying them become narrowed or obstructed. Improving the blood supply to the joints by regular active exercise and healthy food helps them gradually improve. Also, just as a bridge has a load limit, so do your joints. Do your back, hips, and knees a favor by keeping your weight within normal limits.

Part IV

PROBLEMS WITH DRUGS

The Hockey Player's Gold Mine
Tobacco

Here's Ned Walker's story in his own words:
In the middle of a hockey game my arm started to hurt. My elbow pad felt tight, so I slid it down. Later, going up some stairs, I felt the tightness again, this time across my chest as well. I blamed it on my cigarettes. After all, I was only 35 years old, quite solidly muscular, and led a very active life. Heart disease happens to older guys, I reassured myself, the ones who sit in stuffy offices and get fat. Most weekends found me riding my bicycle or motorcycle, playing hockey, or working out. How could I have heart trouble?

AFTER SMOKING ONLY THREE WEEKS, I DEVELOPED AN INTENSE CRAVING FOR IT THAT NEVER LEFT.

But my smoking was something else. I knew it was hurting me. I had tried to stop at least 20 times without success. I had started smoking at age 18 because it seemed to be the mature thing to do. After only three weeks of smoking, I developed an intense craving for it that never left. I needed nearly two packs a day to satisfy that craving.

I knew I needed help, but I kept putting it off. I was involved in six major business enterprises and felt I couldn't leave. Last summer I took off for Alaska to work in my gold mine—something I had looked forward to all year. But I couldn't do much. I was tired all the time, and the pain was almost constant. I finally gave up and decided to come to this health center. If the people here could just help me gain freedom from my cigarette habit, I felt it would be worth the time and money.

When Larry Green, a nurse from the health center, met me at the airport, I still had a pack of cigarettes in my pocket. As we walked to the baggage area, I asked when I was supposed to stop the cigarettes. Larry gave me a long look and replied, "Right now might be a good time." So I tossed the pack in the trash can.

Arriving at the health center an hour later, I was tired and nervous from the long trip and shaky from the lack of a cigarette. Larry must have anticipated this, because he took me directly to hydrotherapy and put me in the Russian steam bath. After sweating things out for a while, I told Larry I felt relaxed and refreshed. I slept well all night.

A few days later, when the tests were finished, the doctors told me I had coronary artery heart disease with a disabling amount of angina. I was shocked, but I was also relieved to know I wasn't a hypochondriac after all.

I adjusted to the food—and even pronounced it OK when I began to see that the simplicity of the food and the modest amount of salt contributed toward decreasing my craving for cigarettes. So did walks in the fresh, brisk air. In fact, when I wanted a cigarette, I would go out for a walk, and the craving would soon dissipate.

And I learned to slow down. I got back in touch with my spiritual nature. As a matter of fact, I had become a born-again Christian six years before, and I wanted to give my life totally to God. I had quit booze, but it bothered me that I couldn't quit those cigarettes.

I thought back on my life. I had been healthy and active until age 27. Then I took on more and more of a businessperson's lifestyle with its stress and poor dietary habits, and this is what happened. I'm glad I still have time to turn my health around.

∞

When Ned returned to his home he changed his lifestyle completely. Besides conquering the tobacco habit, he severed himself from four of his six businesses. His life became much less hectic and pressured.

"I can honestly say I feel as I did in my 20s—no, actually as I did in my teens, before I started smoking," he says now. "I wake up each morning with a clear mind and a zest for a new day. But I do have one problem—now I'm hooked on peanut butter! Do you have a cure for that?" He grins.

Ned's father and grandfather both died of heart disease in their early 40s. Excited by his new knowledge of how to avoid such an outcome, Ned returned to the health center several months later, bringing his sister and his aunt and uncle to the live-in health program. He looked tan, relaxed, fit, happy—quite a contrast to the serious, pale, tense, depressed man we'd seen six months before.

"You know," he reflected, "I discovered a

much better gold mine here than the one I have in Alaska! Really!"

Recent findings suggest that the risk of lung cancer from smoking relates less to the total years smoked than to the age at which smoking began. A young person, it appears, is more likely to sustain permanent DNA damage.

I Was a Coffee Addict
Caffeine

A long with almost everyone else, I didn't believe coffee was addictive. But most coffee contains caffeine, and, like other mood-enhancing drugs, caffeine quietly sinks its tentacles into many of our bodies.

When I joined a health seminar my first battle entailed trying to quit coffee. The first five days were some of the most miserable in my life. My head ached incessantly. I was too nauseated to eat. Then I was too weak to walk. Twice I was at the end of my endurance and ready to quit. But the doctor urged me to hang on a little longer. On the fifth day the symptoms cleared, and I started feeling really good.

I DIDN'T BELIEVE COFFEE WAS ADDICTIVE.

I had no idea that coffee could do this to a person. How I had longed for just one cup! But I was glad I was allowed to suffer. The experience is indelibly etched in my memory. Whenever I smell it, whenever I feel the tiniest temptation, the memories come flooding back, and I won't touch it. This is the best kind of affirmative action.

∞

Not everyone's withdrawal is as difficult as was Betty's. But nearly everyone suffers some degree of headache and lassitude the first few days after quitting caffeinated drinks. A person can get hooked with a relatively small amount of caffeine if it's taken on a fairly regular basis.

Every day eight of 10 people in North America take in caffeine, the world's most popular psychotropic (mind-altering) drug—and coffee isn't the only culprit. Caffeine is added to most colas, Dr. Pepper, some orange sodas, and other soft drinks. Six of the seven most popular soft drinks contain caffeine.

Caffeine is also an ingredient in an array of everyday foods and drugs—brewed and iced teas, many painkillers and headache remedies, some allergy and sinus medications, some weight control pills—more than 1,000 over-the-counter and prescription drugs.

On a body/weight basis, children ages 1 to 5 years are the heaviest consumers of caffeine—mostly from chocolate and sodas. One can of a caffeinated soda in a small child is equivalent to four cups of coffee in an average-sized adult. Pepsi, 7-Up, and Dr. Pepper have licensed their logos to major makers of baby bottles. Parents are four times more likely to give their children soda pop when their kids use these logo bottles than when they don't.

Commercials for products high in caffeine appeal to

teens who are looking for legal drugs that act as stimulants. But using a chemical to "feel good" is a behavior that may serve as a gateway to the use of other drugs.

Caffeine does heighten alertness and mask fatigue—but at a price. It's not a lift without a letdown. Caffeine can produce irregular heartbeat, increased blood pressure, elevated blood sugar, increased stomach acid production, insomnia, tremors, irritability, and nervousness. Caffeine has also been shown to precipitate asthma attacks, anxiety and panic disorders, and to heighten symptoms of PMS.

In spite of its common use, caffeine is just another bad habit. Choose to live drug-free. Choose health!

FEELING TIRED?

You may be dehydrated. Your body needs six to eight glasses of water every day. In fact, since caffeine pulls water *out* of your system, every time you have a caffeinated drink you need to back it up with extra water. Keep your body hydrated, and it may chase away that tired feeling.

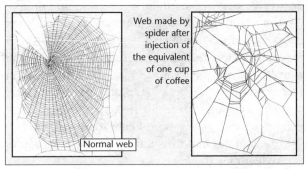

A Spider's Web, Witt, P. N., et al., Springer-Verlag New York, Inc., 1968, fig 9, p. 30 and fig. 25, p. 61. © Springer-Verlag GmbH & Co. KG. Used by permission.

The Robot Awakens

Prescription Medications

"For nearly two years I've been walking around in a daze, feeling like a robot," Jean said. "I can't take it anymore. I've gotten so depressed I hardly care to live." Her tired, listless eyes contrasted sharply with her attractive, youthful appearance and her stylish clothes. I probed to discover her problem.

"I was pretty much OK until two years ago, when I began feeling stressed and tired and had trouble sleeping. My physical checkup was essentially OK except for an elevated blood pressure. To take care of that my doctor started me on medications, and now I'm taking eight different kinds."

"For your blood pressure?"

"Let's see. I think three are for my blood pressure, one is to calm my nerves, and two others help me sleep—" She stopped, suddenly self-conscious, and shifted her focus. "Nothing helped; in fact, I felt worse. Finally I became so upset that I threw them all out and quit, cold turkey. But my blood pressure went up again, and the doctor told me sternly that those medications must be taken for life, and I had better make up my mind to it.

"I feel trapped in a life I hate, but I see no way out." Her eyes were pleading now. "I have a won-

> *I FELT TRAPPED IN A LIFE I HATED. I TRULY BELIEVED MY VERY SURVIVAL DEPENDED ON MY MEDICATIONS.*

derful husband, but I'm no longer an adequate wife."
She looked away, blinking hard.

I took her hands in mine. "Look at me, Jean,"
I commanded. "God sent you here, and we can
help you!"

A small smile began to tug at her face. "Actually,
my uncle sent me here," she corrected. "But I know
I'm grasping at a straw, and I'm scared to death. I
guess I do need God." She sat on the edge of her
chair, opening and closing her hands as we began talking about her treatment.

"Jean, do you realize the length of your depression
coincides almost exactly with the length of time you've
been on heavy medication? How do you feel about
slowly cutting down the dosages while you are here?"

Jean froze, panic and terror in her eyes. She was
right. She was scared to death. She truly believed that
her very survival depended on those medications.

I backed off. "OK; let's compromise. You pick
out one of the blood pressure medications, and we'll
reduce the dose just a little bit. We'll watch you carefully, monitor your blood pressure, and restore the
dose if anything happens."

Jean gradually settled into the program. She was
introduced to foods low in sugar, salt, and fat, but
high in fiber, vitamins, minerals, colors, and textures.
And she was introduced to miles of beautiful trails on
which to walk. She learned how to lose weight and
enjoyed the sunbaths. She drank gallons of water. Day
by day her confidence increased and her medication
doses shrank. She walked between five and six miles a
day and lost 13 pounds. Her blood cholesterol

dropped an astounding 93 points, from 278 mg/dl (7.1 mmol/l) to 185 (4.8).

By the last 10 days of the program Jean was off all medications, including her three blood pressure pills. Even so, her blood pressure remained right around 120/80. Jean purchased her own blood pressure equipment so she could check it for herself.

Wondering what was going on, Jean's husband flew down from Canada to check things out. He was trim, fit, friendly, and very handsome—every bit the prize Jean had described. "I can't believe what I'm seeing!" he exclaimed. "Is this vital, alert, gorgeous woman really my wife?"

"You bet I am!" Jean shot back, as they hugged each other. "This robot woke up and walked back into reality."

∽

Of course, not everyone responds quite as dramatically as Jean did. Not everyone with high blood pressure can get off medication. Medicines obviously have their place but should generally be a last resort, because there are always side effects. In Jean's case, her medications nearly ruined her life.

Part V

THOSE GOLDEN YEARS

The Incredible Hiking Hulda
How Old Is Old?

Newspaper headlines around the world reported her triumphs. Reporters from television, radio stations, and newspapers vied for interviews and took pictures. Her telephone rang and rang.

Who was this media darling of the late 1980s? A quiet, gentle old woman named Hulda Crooks. Barely five feet tall, with hair like a puff of snow, she became a celebrity all because of her unique quest for health.

"BETTER TO FALL GASPING ON THE TRAIL THAN ADMIT YOU'VE BEEN DONE IN BY CHEESEBURGERS AND PIZZA."

How did it happen? Very slowly, actually. Hardly anyone had ever heard of her until she started climbing Mount Whitney at age 66. For the next 25 years she kept climbing that 14,494-foot peak. She reached the top 23 times and was prevented from completing the hike only twice, because of severe weather and poor trail conditions.

Hulda did not start life as a robust child. She recalls those early days and admits to problems with overeating. "I would eat chocolate until I threw up, and then I would eat some more. My brother told me I was going to be as wide as I was tall."

Instead she studied dietetics and adopted the vegetarian lifestyle. She married, had a son, kept house, and tended her garden, her flowers, and her animals. Her life might have continued in peaceful anonymity except that before she was 65 she had lost her husband and her only child.

Alone and lonely, she longed for a challenge and for a way to share her faith. She loved mountains and had often dreamed of climbing some of the great peaks. So she began walking. As her strength increased, so did her adventures. At a time when most women are relaxing into comfortable retirement, Hulda began conquering mountains.

I met Hulda Crooks in 1986, when she was 90 years old. She told me that several months before her yearly Whitney climb she had teasingly challenged Congressman Jerry Lewis of California's thirty-fifth district to "climb the mountain with me next time." She said it in fun, never dreaming he would actually accept.

But the challenge was hard to refuse: climb Mount Whitney, the tallest peak in the contiguous United States, with 90-year-old Hulda Crooks. Was she implying that he might not be able to keep up? How could he let this gutsy little great-grandmother, nearly twice his age, get away with that?

So Mr. Lewis embarked on a serious conditioning program. On the morning of the climb he looked trim, fit, and he was 30 pounds lighter. Later, standing atop Mount Whitney, he sported a T-shirt that proclaimed "By Hook or by Crooks."

"I'm a new man," he announced.

The Whitney climb is no afternoon pleasure

jaunt. Reporter Steve Cooper described it this way: "Above the 12,000-foot level, although a few athletes stroll by looking superior, most folks are sweating, sucking oxygen with the force of an industrial vacuum cleaner, and feeling their legs turn to rubber. Altitude sickness can strike with its double-you-over nausea and a headache that comes on like a freight train. The sensible thing would be to hike back down to where the air is.

HEALTH IS YOUR PRIZE FOR LIVING IN HARMONY WITH THE LAWS ESTABLISHED BY YOUR CREATOR.

"But turning tail would be an excruciating embarrassment if you are walking with this incredibly strong 90-year-old vegetarian. Better to fall gasping on the trail than to admit you've been done in by cheeseburgers and pizza."

You are the oldest known person to have reached the 14,494-foot summit of Mount Whitney reads a plaque awarded Hulda by the U.S. Department of Agriculture. She also held nine national records for women more than 80 years old in the quarter and half marathons, as well as in the 10-kilometer run. Her exploits found their way into national newspapers, magazines, network television, health films, and even into the *Congressional Record*.

Even so, Hulda shunned the limelight. Continued Cooper, "She is a teacher and a gentle conscience in the midst of a society conspicuous for its overconsumption and sedentary living. She wishes to use her mountain fame only as a means to have her message heard."

Zeroing in on today's go-now-pay-later generation, she worried about their obsession with the present and their unawareness of their future health.

"Research indicates that a healthful lifestyle can hold back the aging process as much as 30 years," she pointed out. "Thirty extra years of good health is like an extension of youth. Who could turn down a bargain like that?"

"I want to be like you when I get old," a teenager said admiringly.

"It doesn't come easy," Hulda told her. "You've got to start right now and work for it."

Hulda Crooks was the grandmother everyone dreams of having. Her blue eyes sparkled with fun, her laugh was infectious and disarming, and her grit was as true as her character. A spunky sense of adventure was one of her hallmarks.

In May 1996 Hulda Crooks celebrated her 100th birthday. "Gentle Mountain Tamer Turns 100" announced the San Bernardino *Sun* in bold black letters on the front page of its Sunday news section. Accompanying a full-color picture were these words: "An uncommon woman who scaled lofty mountains and hiked steep canyons, refusing to age humbly."

Hulda Crooks died peacefully in her sleep a year later. To the end she assured everyone, "I'm not waiting around for the Grim Reaper. I'm waiting for the Life-giver."

HULDA'S HEALTH TIPS

• Rich or poor, wise or foolish, we are limited to one body per customer—no exchanges, trade-ins, or replacements. And only one lease on life is granted. The body's performance during that lease is largely dependent on the intelligent care we give to it.

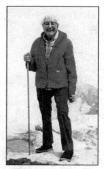

• Muscles that are not used atrophy; bones not put under stress lose minerals and become weak; joints not moved sufficiently, as in walking, working, or other forms of exercise, become stiff from disuse.

• No amount of exotic foods, costly elixirs, vitamins, minerals, or other supplements will save the body from deterioration if your way of life is at fault.

• The Good Book tells us to love God not only with all our strength, but with all our heart, mind, and soul. We need to count the happy moments of each day and be grateful for whatever good comes to us, be it seemingly ever so little.

• There is too much depression, particularly among older people. Talk of things that give joy. Linger over each find with a thankful heart. This will grow into a most rewarding habit. People with a faith in God and hope for the future can go through anything. It's adversity that makes us grow strong.

• It's never too early, and it's also never too late, to get started. Health is your prize for living in harmony with the laws established by your Creator.

• Formula for a healthful lifestyle: Learn to enjoy good food, simply prepared—whole-grain breads and cereals, fresh fruits, vegetables, and legumes, eaten at regular mealtimes. Between meals, drink a quart or more of water each day. Get regular exercise. You don't have to climb mountains or run marathons, but nearly everyone can walk. In fact, recent studies rate walking ahead of nearly every other form of exercise.

My Legs Keep Going

Leg Cramps

It's so frustrating," Mae said with disgust. "I can't walk a block without my legs cramping. Is it expecting too much to want to be active and vital past age 77?"

Age 77? I did a double take. This attractive woman who looked as though she was ready to spill over with fun and energy was 77?

EXERCISE MAY NOT BE A FOUNTAIN OF YOUTH, BUT IT'S THE CLOSEST THING WE HAVE.

She clapped her hand over her mouth. "Now I've gone and done it! I didn't mean to tell you my age! Promise me you won't write it down anywhere." She tried to stare fiercely at me, but started to giggle.

I laughed too. But I knew her request was serious.

"I keep wondering if it's worth the investment to seek further medical help," she continued, composed now. "This place is pretty expensive, you know. I suppose a person has to accept a few discomforts as the years pass." She paused, locking her eyes with mine. "But I *refuse* to accept old age without a fight!"

I loved her spunkiness. "OK; let's fight! Your problem, as you probably know, is poor circulation in your legs. My problem is to find a way to correct your problem."

"You mean operate?" She was suspicious now.

"No, no, not that. Something much more difficult. But I can't do it for you. I'll teach you how, and then it's up to you to do it."

She looked at me quizzically, wondering if I was playing games.

Mae had always considered herself a bit of a health nut. She had never touched alcohol, cigarettes, or even caffeinated beverages. She was also a vegetarian. With all this good living, she couldn't imagine what more could be done for her, short of medications and/or surgery.

"Admit it or not, Mae, you are 77 years old. Your good health and sharp mind reflect your healthy lifestyle, but you need help with those legs.

"You see," I went on, "there are several ways we can get more blood into your legs. One way is to put you on a diet that's very low in fat. Fat thickens the blood, and the red blood cells start sticking to each other, retarding circulation. Cleaning out excess fat from the blood increases circulation almost immediately. Second, hydrotherapy [water] treatments will loosen up your arteries. Heat dilates arteries, and cold constricts at first, then dilates them as the blood tries to warm up the cold area. Your third assignment is exercise. Walk as far as you can, then rest when the cramps start. Do this several times a day. Exercise not only stimulates your remaining circulation but also helps build up collateral circulation."

Encouraged, Mae decided to stay. She loved the water treatments, and she loved walking in the sunshine and fresh air of the Sierra Nevada foothills. Her leg cramps decreased fairly quickly, and after a week she could walk the better part of a mile without pain.

Although she'd been a lifelong vegetarian, she decided to eliminate dairy products and visible fats and oils as well. She took this step toward a *very* low-fat diet because of scientific findings demonstrating that clogged arteries can be cleaned out on such a program.

By the end of the month Mae was walking three miles with minimal pain. She was as happy as a little girl on a merry-go-round. "My daughter is going to be very surprised when we walk through the shopping mall together, because she won't have to stop every two seconds for my leg cramps to go away."

Four years later I met Mae again. She hadn't changed. "I'm having a lot of fun for an old lady," she joked. "And yes, I've stuck to what I learned—at least 90 percent of the time. I'm active, happy, and on the go all day long. I am the Community Services leader at our church. The cramps in my legs have stopped. I enjoy life and feel fine. My only regret is that so few people are open to learning about this lifestyle. Most feel they must get terribly ill before they need to change their lifestyle. But this is such a good life! I praise God for His blessings."

In a recent letter from her I noted with a smile that she is no longer secretive about her age:

"I'm 92 years old now, and, aside from annoying arthritis at times, am enjoying good health. I still carry on most of my usual pursuits, except driving my car, which I prefer not to do in today's busy traffic. I continue to praise God for restoring my health."

One of her nieces told me, with a touch of awe, "Can you believe Aunt Mae goes camping with us? She is so much fun, and she tells us that she honestly doesn't feel a day over 60!"

And she's right! Research indicates that a healthy lifestyle can hold back the aging process as much as 30 years. Today health, rather than years, usually determines one's status. Premature aging and disability are largely the result of lifestyle factors such as smoking, excessive alcohol and caffeine consumption, and the abuse of drugs. Being overweight speeds up physical and sexual decline. A diet of rich, refined foods and lack of regular exercise can make people old before their time.

Old age sets in when disease and disability limit everyday tasks. Some people are old while still relatively young in years. These are usually people who are chronically ill, injured, or victims of a major tragedy, many of whom withdraw and give up on life. Others remain youthful and vital, interesting and productive into advanced age, as Mae so well demonstrates.

Reaching a Little Higher

Asthma

Death Valley's debilitating heat sucked Richard Kegley's strength as he stepped from the cool desert museum into the 111° outdoor heat. He was about to begin one of the world's toughest challenges to runners: the Death Valley to Mount Whitney run. The rules required that he run the distance between the lowest (282 feet below sea level) and highest

(14,494 feet) points in the contiguous United States during the peak of summer, between July 1 and August 31. The 146-mile run would take him from the scorching desert heat to near freezing temperatures atop Mount Whitney.

Richard knew that only eight of the 80 people before him who had officially attempted this course during the previous 10 years had finished. And the oldest of the eight had been 10 years younger than he was.

Here it is, he thought. *The first step, the step that's going to commit me to this ordeal.*

It was hot, so very hot.

I can't even breathe—how can I run? He almost panicked. *Put one foot down, then the next. Again. Again.*

Soon he was in rhythm. The sliver of moon seemed out of place in the oppressive heat. He looked up at the stars shimmering beyond the hot air and thought about how he had gotten from a hospital bed 10 years before, clutching an oxygen mask, to this punishing run in Death Valley.

AH, BUT A MAN'S REACH SHOULD EXCEED HIS GRASP, OR WHAT'S A HEAVEN FOR?
—ROBERT BROWNING.

Death Valley, that's what his life had been. Richard had suffered from asthma for years. Even though he carried a small pharmacy with him, he had frequent flare-ups that repeatedly landed him in the hospital. After his last admission at age 58, he decided he had to do something different. He had a few things going for him. He didn't smoke or drink, and he had been a vegetarian all his life. But in spite of all that clean living, he had put on an extra 50 pounds. And there was that asthma.

He bought an exercise bicycle and began to use it every day. His doctor son prescribed a regimen of walking. Soon he was walking the two miles to his auto dealership. His wife, Margaret, joined him. She had her own problems, having survived a stroke and four heart attacks, as well as being overweight. They now cut all refined foods and most sugars, fats, and animal foods from their diet.

Within a month Richard ran a mile. Within a few more months Margaret had dropped 20 pounds and had run her first marathon, placing second in her age group. As Richard's endurance improved, the extra weight disappeared. His asthma faded away and never returned. He began to enjoy life. He felt young again. By this time he and Margaret were both hooked on running. Margaret covered two to four miles, and Richard six to eight miles, five days a week. They both ran marathons.

During the next 10 years Richard ran 25,000 miles. His credits include the Boston Marathon, four Lake Tahoe runs (72 miles each), and four Six-Day races in San Diego. In the 1984 Six-Day Race he set a new record for men older than 60 by covering 331 miles. But tonight, in the oppressive heat of Death Valley, those distant successes seemed like faded dreams. The cloying heat, the 180-degree ground temperature, the desperate barrenness that gave Death Valley its name, settled upon him and penetrated to the core. But he would keep going. *Put one foot down, then the other, again, again.*

He didn't want to fail. And he didn't. On the fifth day of the run he became, at age 68, the oldest person at that time to complete the Death Valley-Mount Whitney run. He was a winner!

But Richard had been a victor long before this. He had salvaged what had been the wreck of his physical self. He had faced overwhelming odds. It didn't happen all at once. He took one step, then another, again, again, year after year. And he won the most important battle—the battle for his health.

Richard and Margaret are now in their late 70s. It's been more than 20 years since Richard has had an asthma attack. In fact, they both felt so good that they ran the Portland Marathon together to celebrate their golden wedding anniversary.

I'm Tired of Colonics

Constipation

"I'm not really sure why I'm here," Mildred said. "Probably because it's my last hope. After all, I'm 79 years old, and you have to die sometime." Her ample body slumped into her chair as dejection etched the lines of her face.

> I GO FOR COLONIC IRRIGATIONS TWICE A WEEK TO ELIMINATE PROPERLY.

"My life is a mess," she continued. "My digestion is poor—I've been eating six small meals a day and still feel bloated. I have to go for colonic irrigations twice a week to eliminate properly. My blood pressure is too high, and my circulation is so poor that my ankles are swollen and discolored. I'm much too heavy. I'm taking 11 different medications, but they don't seem to do any good. I just feel so miserable that I told my daughter I didn't think I wanted to live much longer. She persuaded me to come here, but I don't think much can be done for my condition."

She looked so forlorn that I leaned forward and took her hands in mine. "Your condition isn't so hopeless," I assured her with a cheery smile. "Let me tell you about some of the things we can do for you."

She straightened up and a glimmer of hope glinted her eyes.

"For one thing, your diet here will be largely full-fiber plant foods. Fiber is the framework of plants, but because fiber is not absorbed into the body, people believed it was useless. Removing this 'useless' fiber was thought to improve the value of food and make it easier to digest."

I explained to her that now we know fiber is valuable, acting as a kind of general, controlling many body processes. For example:

• Insoluble fiber absorbs and holds water—up to six times its own volume—creating soft, spongy masses in the stomach and intestines. The result? A sense of fullness occurs much sooner than with low-fiber foods, helping to protect against overeating and obesity.

• The fiber masses, acting like soaked-up sponges, fill the intestines more completely and stimulate them to lively activity. Instead of taking several days to go through the gastrointestinal tract in compacted lumps, as low-fiber foods do, the spongy masses pass along much more quickly and are evacuated in 24 to 36 hours. Faster elimination cures most constipation and significantly relieves problems with hemorrhoids and diverticular disease.

• Fiber slows down the rate at which foods enter the bloodstream. This helps smooth out the ups and downs of blood sugar levels and provides more consistent energy throughout the day. A stabilized blood sugar relieves most hypoglycemia [low blood sugar] and aids in the control of diabetes [high blood sugar].

• Fiber helps protect the colon from cancer.

"We don't use processed and refined foods at our health center because they have little or no fiber, and meat and dairy products have no fiber at all."

"But won't all that 'roughage' bother my stomach?" Mildred asked.

"No, it won't, because in the body, fiber becomes soft. What will help your stomach is spacing your meals four to five hours apart, giving it time to digest each meal thoroughly. Your food will also have very little salt, which helps pull out extra water your body is holding. When that happens, your blood pressure and your swollen ankles will improve. You must also walk outdoors every day. This helps you lose weight and chases away your stress and depression."

"Are you *sure?*" Mildred was dubious. "All that sounds too good to be true."

Despite her doubts, Mildred gamely plunged into her routine without complaints. But I still worried about those twice weekly colonic irrigations she was accustomed to having. We didn't give those treatments at our center, and I wondered how patient she would be about waiting for her normal elimination to catch up. Many older people become obsessed with their bowels. If they miss a day they are convinced that poisons will begin creeping into their bodies. My assurances that some people go for weeks without elimination with no ill effects usually fall on deaf ears.

My concern evaporated when Mildred happily reported "results" the third day. Miserable or not, she was giving the program her best effort. Three weeks later we were again in my office. This time, however, Mildred was all smiles, her eyes bright and alive.

"I've changed my mind about my condition," she reported. "So far I've lost 13 pounds. I'm eating three meals a day with good appetite and have no more digestive problems. I've not needed a single colonic irrigation. My blood pressure has come down, and the swelling in my legs is nearly gone. I need only three medications a day now." She paused, then added with conviction, "But the best thing is my mental outlook. I feel so much better now that my problems don't seem so serious. I feel like I'm in control of my life again. Sure, I feel lonely, and I still have trouble sleeping. But I don't want to die anymore. I've got too much to live for. I can't wait to get home."

What Follows the Swallows?

Snacks, Indigestion

I'm not sure what's wrong, but I just don't feel good," Margaret Mason told me. "It all began with a new job about a year ago. The stressful work, the cranky boss, the gossipy coworkers, along with all the problems at home, just seemed to sap my energy. I began drinking extra cups of coffee and more colas to combat the fatigue.

"It wasn't long before my stomach became so irritated that I no longer enjoyed my meals. My doctor prescribed antacid medications, which didn't help. I tried several small meals a day, but that upset my digestion. I feel bloated all the time. Do you think I have an ulcer?"

MOST PEOPLE CHOOSE TO QUIET THEIR "BUBBLE MACHINE" WITH THE LATEST PHARMACEUTICAL PREPARATIONS.

"Maybe," I answered, "but your symptoms are more likely a result of mistreating your stomach."

"I suppose you're right." Margaret looked at the floor. "I'm sure the coffee and colas aren't helping. Do you think that might be the whole trouble?"

"It's possible, but I doubt it. However, the first step toward recovery is to eliminate those stomach irritants. Coffees contain aromatic oils that can irritate sensitive stomach linings. Coffee, tea, and many soft drinks contain caffeine, which constricts blood vessels and stimulates excessive acid in the stomach. The additives in many beverages are another source of irritants."

"No wonder I'm in trouble," Margaret observed. "Why don't they tell people these things?"

I had to smile. "Do people really want to know? Because these beverages also produce desirable effects, most people choose to quiet their 'bubble machine' with the latest pharmaceutical preparations.

I went on to explain that an even worse problem is the way we abuse our digestive processes. The stomach works best when it receives a meal, has time to break down the food particles to a more uniform size, bring it to the needed consistency and acidity, and send it on into the intestines. Then the stomach needs time to rest a while before the next meal arrives.

In one study a group of students at a large university received a breakfast of cereal, toast, fruit, and an egg. After four hours, their stomachs were empty. A few days later the same students ate the same breakfast, but two hours after eating they were given either a peanut butter sandwich or a piece of pumpkin pie with a glass of milk. Six to nine hours later a part of their breakfast was still in their stomachs.

One person received a little chocolate candy twice in the morning and twice during the afternoon. Some 13 hours later more than half the breakfast was still in the stomach—still undigested.

"You make it sound as though we shouldn't eat any snacks at all!" Margaret exclaimed. "These days *everybody* snacks!"

"And nearly everybody has problems with indigestion, heartburn, irritability, insomnia, mental dullness, or weight gain. A pattern of three meals a day—with no snacking—could solve many of these problems. And meals should be spaced four to five hours apart."

Margaret shrugged. "OK; I'm convinced. I'll give it a try."

"It won't be easy," I cautioned. "But if you stick to it, I guarantee you will feel much better. Drink lots of water between meals. If you must have more food, eat a piece of fresh fruit. I'll see you in two weeks."

When she returned, Margaret was radiant. "After three days my appetite came back and my stomach problems disappeared. What a simple solution! I've been telling all my friends." She paused and looked at me quizzically. "Doctor, why don't you write a book about this."

"I'd like to," I sighed. "But who would believe it?"

NOTE: A pattern of three meals a day, with no snacking, could solve many of the problems of indigestion, heartburn, irritability, insomnia, mental dullness, and weight gain that are plaguing so many people today.

Sweetheart of the Marathon
Motivation

Tiny Mavis Lindgren is a celebrity in her own right. Tired of being a pulmonary cripple with frequent hospitalizations for pneumonia, she began training at age 70. By age 85 she had run 63 marathons. I met her just after she'd turned 89. She had already run three marathons that year and was itching to do another one.

"What I'd really like to do next is run the London Marathon," she confided. "If

"AT AGE 89 IT'S A WONDERFUL THING TO GET UP IN THE MORNING AND NOT HURT ANYWHERE."
—MAVIS LINDGREN, MARATHON RUNNER

I succeed, do you think I might get to meet Queen Elizabeth?"

That's the secret ingredient of people like Mavis Lindgren—they take each day a step at a time, but they never run out of dreams!

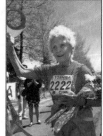

Mavis Lindgren

> It's a calamity to die
> With dreams unfulfilled, but
> It is a calamity not to dream.
> —*Benjamin E. Mays*

Part VI

FORMING HABITS

Children at Risk

It's Never Too Early

My plans to stay home with my little son blew up one day, and I needed day care. I did extensive research in the area where I live, looking for a place that had loving and conscientious people and also a good nutritional program. I finally found one that seemed right. They had a garden of organic vegetables. Kids worked in the garden, picking and preparing the vegetables. They even made zucchini bread on occasion.

I'M SO GLAD WE MADE THE DECISION TO EMPHASIZE RIGHT NUTRITION AS PART OF OUR SON'S EARLY LIFE.

When I took 2½-year-old Aidan for his test day, I was pleased to see all the kids sit down for a meal of kasha, zucchini squash, beet greens, tofu, and almonds, topped off with soy milk. About three hours later I called the center to see how Aidan was doing. Karen, the assistant, answered the phone and gushed, "Oh, he's amazing! He's unbelievable! No kid does this the first day."

What was this woman talking about? What did my son do? At least it sounded as though something good was happening. Then the school's director came on the line. "Do you know what Karen is talking about?" I asked her.

"Oh!" she laughed. "All the teachers are amazed because Aidan ate everything on his plate, and they've never seen that happen before to a new student on the first day." She added, "I can always tell which kids are brought up with good wholesome nutrition. They immediately take to the food, while most children take weeks, even months, to adjust to our natural diet."

That gave me validation for what we had been doing with Aidan's nutrition. Aidan not only eats great food; he also helps pick it out in the market. Then he helps in the preparation and cooking. He is involved with his food, and that encourages healthy eating habits.

It's not easy taking the high road and emphasizing natural foods. It is also expensive and time-consuming. Yet the rewards are obvious. He has a healthy immune system and an appreciation for good food. As I watch other moms and dads struggle to get their kids to eat healthy foods, I'm so glad that we made the decision to emphasize right nutrition as part of his early life.

∞

One day, instead of serving the usual hot meal, the school cafeteria handed out peanut-butter-and-jelly sandwiches. After lunch a satisfied first grader marched out the door and complimented the cafeteria manager, "Finally, you gave us a home-cooked meal!"

Sad to say, home-cooked, sitting-down-around-the-table meals are now the exception in most American homes, being largely replaced by fast foods and engineered foods. More than half of today's high school kids head off to fast-food chains and snack machines instead of school lunchrooms. And we are paying the price. "Heart disease begins in childhood," reports the National Institutes of Health. An examination of 360 randomly selected youngsters aged 7 to 12 revealed that 98 percent of the children already had three or more risk factors.

A related problem is that children are getting fatter faster than ever. A recent study found that 22 percent of kids under age 12 are overweight, and the total goes up to 57 percent for teens aged 13 to 17.

Being overweight predisposes a child to heart disease, gallstones, adult-onset diabetes, hypertension, cancer, and full-blown obesity later in life. Obese children have more orthopedic problems and more upper respiratory diseases. And that is only one side of the story. They often suffer major social and psychological problems. The rapid increase of serious depression, eating disorders, drug use, and suicide among teenagers is frightening.

Genes can play a role in a person's weight, but they aren't the whole answer. Environment plays a critically important role, as shown by the fact that the percentage of obese Americans has increased steadily during the past 50 years. Our gene pool can't change that fast!

Another concern is that about 80 percent of overweight teenagers will remain overweight as adults. The increase in adolescent obesity (about 40 percent during the past 15 years) will have serious consequences in the future. Already adult diabetes (Type II), usually considered a disease of middle age and later, is showing up in obese children.

The major causes of obesity in children are the same as for adults—a sedentary lifestyle, TV viewing, the Internet, the snack and soda habit, and the popularity and availability of highly processed and concentrated foods. Many major medical centers are developing weight-control programs for children that involve the whole family. Proper eating and lifestyle habits are a family affair, and a youngster, especially, needs the support of the family. Even when the rest of the family is not overweight, everyone benefits from a healthier way of life.

Saving the child just might save the family.

> "Stay away from junk food, get off the couch, unplug the Nintendo, turn off the TV, and go out and get some exercise. A body is a terrible thing to waste."—Arnold Schwarzenegger.

A Child Shall Lead

Kids as Teachers

Bryan's grandmother made the best Toll House cookies in the world. Like the biblical widow's flask of oil, her cookie jar was never empty. Kids, grandkids, and friends alike anticipated munching those crispy rich delicacies filled with gooey globs of chocolate.

Five-year-old Bryan, especially, loved visiting Grandma. One night after supper and story time

Grandma felt like rewarding Bryan for being such a good boy all day. She offered him a cookie.

"But Grandma," the little boy said earnestly, "I've already brushed my teeth!"

The next morning a somewhat-chastened Grandma tried another strategy. At breakfast she produced a box of Froot Loops—a surefire hit with any kid, especially one who was growing up on "health foods" at home.

This time Bryan's voice dripped reproach. "Grandma!" he exclaimed. "Do you want me to get holes in my teeth?"

Grandma remembered something in the Bible about training a child right (Proverbs 22:6). *I guess 5 years old is not too early to start,* she reflected. It's this grandma that needs to "get with it"!

‍꙳

Yes, the good news is that children can be taught—and the younger they get started, the better. Here are some tips for building good health habits early in life:

• Make sure the child gets three meals a day, at regular times, with lots of whole grains, fruits, and vegetables.

• Discourage snacks, and the child will have a better appetite for nutritious food at mealtimes. If a snack is needed, offer a piece of fresh fruit.

• Encourage daily exercise—preferably outdoors—for at least an hour.

• Provide plenty of water. Save sodas for special events.

• Make sure the child gets adequate rest. Most children are chronically tired—not surprising when you remember that teenagers do best on nine hours of sleep each night. Younger ones need more. Put the kids to bed early enough so they awaken naturally in time for a healthy breakfast.

• Control TV. The hours a child watches TV relate directly to weight gain and elevated blood cholesterol levels.

• Cultivate a wide range of interests—schedule library visits, music lessons, arts and crafts, hobbies, and family outings. Children who spend time with their parents and develop deep spiritual roots experience less stress and improved mental health.

• Set a good example. The life choices you are modeling day by day are the strongest determinants of your children's future behavior.

Jumpstart Your Day
Breakfast Power

Five-year-old Christy munched solemnly on half a breakfast sweet roll. Her mother, father, grandfather, and I, lounging on beds and chairs, were doing likewise. We were vacationing together, sharing transportation as well as motel rooms. This day we thought we'd hit the jackpot—not only an especially nice room, but free room-delivered Continental breakfasts! Who could resist?

Christy laid her roll on the table and surveyed the rest of us. "Why are we sitting here eating this junk?" Her words were edged with disgust.

Why, indeed? Our reasons withered into feebleness. The morning spread lost its appeal, and we headed out for a "real" breakfast.

∞

Sugar in the morning? You bet! Millions of us start the day with dessert, whether it's sweet rolls, doughnuts, frosted Pop-Tarts, marshmallow-laden cereal, chocolate yogurt, or a muffin the size of a small TV.

Other people can't face food when they crawl out of bed. A quick cup of coffee or a glass of juice is a standard adult breakfast for many. An increasing number of children arrive at school having eaten nothing at all.

"WHY ARE WE SITTING HERE EATING THIS JUNK?"

A sweet roll and a glass of juice are hardly a good breakfast. We need something more substantial, something with more fiber in it. Foods without fiber (especially sugared food and drinks) digest rapidly, leave the stomach, and enter the bloodstream quickly. Up goes the blood sugar, resulting in a quick energy boost—a sugar high.

But the high is only temporary, because it triggers a surge of insulin. Insulin brings down blood sugar levels and, in the absence of the modulating effects of fiber, sometimes pulls it down too fast and too far. A falling blood sugar often mimics symptoms of hypoglycemia, producing feelings of weakness, hunger, fatigue, and letdown—the sugar blues. The usual reaction is to reach for *another* sugary snack, which has led to the now nearly universal morning coffee break.

Although insoluble fiber in food is not digested by the body, it does absorb water as it moves through the stomach and intestines. The resulting spongy mass acts as a gentle barrier to the food particles suspended in it so they are absorbed more gradually. Thus fiber in food slows down the absorption of sugar into the bloodstream. As a result, the sugar levels won't jump around so much, energy is stabilized, and people feel satisfied longer.

A healthful high-fiber breakfast is one that provides at least one third of the day's calories. If you start the day with a whole-grain hot cereal, whole-grain bread, and a couple whole, fresh fruits, you'll find that your energy level stays high throughout the morning.

In the Iowa Breakfast Study a group of scientists spent several years studying the effects of different kinds of breakfasts versus no breakfast at all on people of different ages. A good breakfast, they concluded, can help both children and adults be less irritable, more efficient, and more energetic. Breakfast helped children score higher on tests written during the morning. The steady influx of energy apparently stabilized glucose levels in the brain, improving mental function and attention spans. Other studies, such as the Alameda Study, have even linked healthy breakfasts with less chronic disease, increased longevity, and better health.

Put your children (and yourself) to bed early enough to wake up in time to join the family around

	Calories	fat (gm)	Salt (mg)	Chol. (mg)
BREAKFAST CHOICES				
AMERICAN				
Bacon (3 sl.)	129	12	574	60
Scrambled Eggs (3)	330	24	1,230	675
Hash Browns (1 C)	355	18	3,265	0
Danish Roll (1)	274	15	595	35
Hot Cocoa (1 C)	213	9	295	25
Orange Juice (1 C)	120	0	6	0
TOTAL	**1,421**	**78**	**5,965**	**795**
OPTIMAL				
7-Grain Cereal (1 C)	159	1	400	0
Banana (1)	95	0	3	0
NF Milk/Soy Milk (1 C)	88	0	318	0
Grapefruit (½)	66	0	5	0
Tofu (1 C)	118	7	1,233	0
H. Browns, no oil (1 C)	101	0	22	0
W. W. Bread (1 sl.)	61	1	330	0
TOTAL	**688**	**9**	**2,311**	**0**

the breakfast table. See for yourself the difference it makes. Food is fuel. The brain cells have no stored blood sugar—no energy reserves. Many people are needlessly fatigued because they're not eating early in the day.

The bottom line? A good breakfast boosts your energy, increases your attention span, and heightens your sense of well-being. You'll be less apt to cheat on your diet by snacking. And you'll be in better control of your emotions.

What a great way to start your day!

Orange juice may be nutritious, but it's not as good as the original orange. Orange juice, after all, is defibered orange. The whole fruit, when compared to a cup of juice, requires less insulin to assimilate, lowers cholesterol more effectively, provides smoother digestion with longer appetite satisfaction, and has fewer calories.

A Grandfather's Reward

Snacks

While I was in Singapore recently, Pastor C. D. Chun, president of a large religious organization, told me this story:

My two young grandsons visited us from Seoul, Korea, this past Christmas and New Year season. Because we live so far from them and miss them so much, it was a special joy to be together for more than two weeks. Little Choom is 2 years old, and his brother, Chan, is nearly 5. They are cute, active, and healthy. At each meal they practically emptied every dish on the table. They especially liked the tropical fruit.

MANY CHILDREN GET MORE CALORIES IN THEIR SNACKS IN A DAY THAN THEY DO FROM THEIR MEALS.

It wasn't hard to see the reason they enjoyed their food so much. They were not given any kind of food between meals. In fact, they hardly knew what candy and ice cream were because from the beginning they had not been given such foods. As a result, they enjoyed the wholesome things provided by their mother and grandmother.

On Christmas Day we all went to Jurong Bird Park. I saw a mother urging her young child to finish his lunch. After a few bites, he ran off. Carrying the dish and spoon, the poor mother ran after him, trying to feed him. When children eat sweets and other foods between meals, they have no appetite or desire for wholesome foods at mealtimes. I thought about how carefully we had trained our daughter when she was a child. Now, years later, she is bringing up her own little boys in the same careful way, with the same good habits.

Scientists will say that good health habits are not inherited, but I can tell you from experience that they do pass from one generation to another!

❧

Actually, the idea isn't too surprising. More than 2,000 years ago King Solomon noted in one of his proverbs: "Train up a child in the way he should go, and when he is old, he will not depart from it" (Proverbs 22:6).

But that isn't today's message. Commercials constantly push the idea that we need some kind of energy lift between meals. From birth kids are fed almost constantly. Studies have shown that many children get more calories in a day from their nutrient-poor snacks than they do from their meals.

The same holds true for grown-ups. Fill up on doughnuts, coffee, sodas, and potato chips, and you're going to pass up thousands of the cancer-fighting substances found in fruits and vegetables. Let's face it: most snacks are junk food anyway—candy bars, pork rinds, popcorn, cheese, chocolate-chip cookies, Twinkies, ice cream, and crackers. Often the calories gained from snacks and beverages can add up to more calories than some people should eat *all day!* Is it any wonder we are the fattest nation on earth?

The reason people feel they need snacks is that they eat fiber-poor, sugar-rich meals, without enough complex carbohydrates (starches) and fiber. These "meals" are digested quickly, and the sugars rush into the bloodstream, providing a temporary high. But it doesn't hold for long, and when the blood sugar drops, there is that weak, all-gone feeling that cries for a snack.

Start the day with a whole-grain cereal, whole-wheat bread, and a couple whole fresh fruits, and energy will remain steady all morning. A similar high complex-carbohydrate, high-fiber lunch will do the same for the afternoon. If more is needed, eat a piece

CALORIES FROM SNACKS AND BEVERAGES		
Mid-Morning	Coffee with cream and sugar	75
	Jelly doughnut	255
Mid-Afternoon	Soft drink	140
	Candy bar	295
Late Afternoon	Coffee with cream and sugar	75
	Cookies (3)	350
TV Snack	Soft drink	140
	Potato chips (10)	125
	Cheese crackers (5)	90
	TOTAL	**1,545**

of fresh fruit or a handful of raw veggies. And drink a glass of water.

The snack habit is just that—a habit. When children (and adults) get nourishing, well-balanced meals, there will be much less need for snacks. And appetites will be much improved at mealtimes.

The New Fanatics

Vegetarians

Grandma, is this a real hot dog?" Megan asked when she saw the corn dog on her plate.

We were eating in the Loma Linda University cafeteria, and I assured her that no meat was served in that place.

But Megan was cautious. She looked at her salad. "Grandma, are you sure these aren't real baco bits?"

I again assured her that all was OK, but perhaps there was a touch of impatience in my voice.

Megan lifted her serious 4-year-old eyes and looked straight into mine. "I need to be careful, Grandma," she said solemnly. "I have never eaten any meat in my life, and I don't ever want to. So when I'm not home, I need to ask."

> IN A LIFETIME THE AVERAGE AMERICAN MEAT EATER SUBSIDIZES THE KILLING OF 2,480 CHICKENS, 98 TURKEYS, 32 PIGS AND SHEEP, AND 12 COWS.

115

Megan is right on. Nutritional research confirms that people who don't eat animal products have greater longevity, fewer heart attacks and strokes, fewer weight problems, lower cholesterol, lower blood pressure, and less diabetes. They have less cancer of the breast, prostate, and colon, and fewer hemorrhoids. They also have fewer stones of the kidney and gallbladder, less kidney disease, and less gouty arthritis. Their bones are stronger, and they have less osteoporosis.

Today the "Garden of Eden" diet (Genesis 1:29) is *in*. On every side we are urged to eat more fruits, vegetables, and grains because they contain "phyto-chemicals" and "antioxidants" and fiber—substances the body needs to protect itself from cancer and other serious health threats. The trouble is, while the human body is able to nourish itself on animal foods, it lacks the protection against large amounts of fat and cholesterol that carnivorous animals have. So excessive fat and cholesterol stack up in the bloodstream. Gradually, over time, arteries thicken and narrow, and plaque forms. As a result, blood supplies to vital organs diminish or get cut off and the stage is set for many of today's killer diseases.

The food fanatics of yesteryear have now become today's trendsetters. Whether CEO, lawyer, tennis champion, or homemaker, vegetarians are widely respected. Vegetarianism is increasingly viewed as being smart, healthful, caring, and it leaves a softer footprint on the earth. It's a responsible choice.

Set in Concrete

Can't Change

Y ou know how Ben's belly hangs out over his belt? Well, it's getting worse!"

That piece of conversation might have been a laugh line except that Pat was talking about her husband, and this was not a good omen.

"Is his blood pressure up again?" I wasn't Ben's doctor, but Pat was one of my best friends.

"Probably is, but he hasn't let me check it since he quit his medication." Worry lines creased Pat's face. "The pills make him feel so tired—he says he can't stand it. His doctor has tried several different kinds, but they all make him feel tired."

Ben, an electrician and part-time contractor, was active and energetic. He usually worked at least two jobs at a time.

"And I venture to guess he's also sick and tired of hearing about his weight." I knew that Pat cooked healthful food for her family, but Ben was strictly a meat and potatoes man. With lots of gravy. He wouldn't touch anything else except peas and an occasional salad.

"Things changed for a while last Christmas," Pat continued. "Remember when Ben went to buy a new suit, and the salesclerk brought him a *portly* size? He was so mad he stomped out of the store." Pat smiled at the memory.

"At least it got him back on his program. I remember he'd lost 20 pounds by Easter, and he looked and felt good. What happened?"

"The same old story. He just won't eat the right kind of food, so he is constantly starving. When he can't stand it any longer, he binges. Look at him now—bigger than ever."

I could feel Pat's frustration. It was an ongoing problem that never seemed to get solved.

Pat was teary-eyed. "Ben knows he is eating himself into an early grave, and he hates himself for his weakness. But somewhere early in life his dietary habits got set in concrete."

I wanted to encourage her. "At least he doesn't smoke or drink. And his work gives him plenty of outdoor exercise. He has those things in his favor."

"He must have a pretty strong heart, too," Pat added. "At least he's never had angina."

Sadly, at age 55 Ben had a sudden massive heart attack. He wasn't expected to live, but he survived. For a year he sat at home, tethered to an oxygen tank, reading books and puttering around in his tool shed.

When Ben got stronger, he and Pat packed up their Airstream trailer and joined a group of volunteer church builders. Ben could at least supervise some of the electrical work. "I haven't gone overseas," he would tell his friends, "but I feel like a missionary."

Ben continued to help in this way until a second heart attack ended his life at age 59. His widow and children carry on. And yes, his diet remained set in concrete to the end.

The Three-Week Cure

Can Change

Tanya slumped into her chair with a deep sigh. "Doctor, I'm stuck in a rut." Her voice dripped with weariness. "I want to be healthy, but I snack too much. I don't exercise enough. I drink too much coffee. I'm tired all the time, and I can't seem to change."

"You aren't alone, Tanya," I assured her. "Habits are just about the hardest things in the world to change, because our lifestyles are largely made up of the sum total of our habits. They become part of our identity. The good part is that habits can oil the machinery of our lives, helping us glide through our days, saving time and energy. For example, who would want to have to stop and *think* how to tie a pair of shoelaces? But habits can also make our lives more difficult as well, as you've discovered. Even such a simple act as changing sides of the bed with your spouse can make you uncomfortable."

BY CHOOSING OUR HABITS WE DETERMINE THE GROOVES INTO WHICH TIME WILL WEAR US.

Tanya leaned forward, interested now. "So how do habits form, anyway? And how do we get so stuck in them?"

"Our brains, as you know, were created to serve as headquarters for what goes on in our lives. The brain sends messages to the rest of the body through nerve cells. Each nerve cell has a central processing area and a long sending fiber, called an axon, over which it relays

119

messages. Nerve cells also have lots of tiny receiving fibers, called dendrites, for incoming messages.

"Frequently used axons form tiny bumps. Scientists call these bumps boutons, from the French word for buttons. And the more boutons a nerve cell has, the more easily and quickly it's able to transmit messages."

"OK!" Tanya exclaimed, eyes brightening. "So when we do something again and again is it like the nerve cells are building little pathways in our brains?"

"That's basically the idea. Any thought or action, repeated over and over, makes it easier to repeat that thought or action. Yes, it's almost as though the repetition wears a groove in the brain, much as repeatedly walking over the same place in a lawn will wear a path in the sod."

Tanya paused, considering this concept. "Once those pathways are formed," she worried, "can they be changed?"

"Boutons, unfortunately, do not go away when they are no longer used. And because the old pathways are still there, the chance of falling back into a bad habit is always present. The classic example of this is the alcoholic 'falling off the wagon.'"

"But people *can* change, can't they?"

"Yes, but only by building new habits that are stronger than the old ones. The new choice must be made repeatedly, again and again."

Tanya drew back a little. "That sounds hard, almost hopeless," she ventured.

"It can seem that way at first. But in time more boutons will appear on the new pathway than on the old one, and the 'path' will wear deeper. It then becomes easier to take the new route, and the new habit is becoming established."

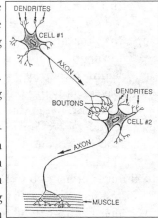

Tanya was tentative. "That must take a long time to happen."

"Sometimes; sometimes not. For instance, a few years ago a woman named Anya Bateman decided to start flossing her teeth. What had been a tiresome chore evolved into a bedtime ritual in less than a month. Encouraged, she applied her three-week plan to breaking her habit of eating too many sweets. Next, she broke her habit of criticizing her husband, then formed a new habit of praising her kids. The results were so astounding that her story was published in *Reader's Digest*."★

"That's the key! I can see it now!" Tanya was getting excited. "I'm always trying to change too many things at once. I need to pick out one new habit and stick with it until those little boutons are formed."

"Yes, that's how it works." I smiled as I watched her despair melt into a surge of hope. "Just as some people become accomplished musicians by many hours of daily practice, we can become a better person by consistently making positive choices. And even if we lose a battle, now and then, we won't lose the war—not as long as we get right back onto that new path we're trying to form."

Tanya sighed happily. "OK, now that I know how to do it, I need to decide where to start." She tapped her foot impatiently.

Knowing that Tanya worried about her weight, I said, "Starting tomorrow, get up a half hour earlier and hit the pavement with a brisk walk or jog. Sure, it may be tough at first, but in three weeks you'll have shed a few pounds, picked up extra energy, gained confidence, and be on your way to a healthier lifestyle."

"All right, I'll do it." The purpose in her voice and the firmness of her step marked a new determination.

"Be sure you check back here in three weeks," I called after her.

---

*Anya Bateman, "Three Weeks to a Better Me," *Reader's Digest,* September 1983.

Failure Is No Big Deal
Trust in God

Angie was coping. Unlike fat, humiliation doesn't show. She chatted easily and laughed often as she made her way through the registration procedures. Underneath her courageous smiling exterior, however, her heart was breaking. She had been a failure. Not just an ordinary failure, but a spectacular one. Failure was not a familiar feeling in her life. Coming back to this place was about the hardest thing she'd ever done.

Angie had been a happy, energetic woman who

breezed through life in high gear. "After all," she told Ted, her husband, "I've outlived Mama and Grandma by a good 10 years. They both died early of heart disease, but I feel just fine."

But Angie wasn't "just fine." One day, flat on her back from an injury, she finally faced reality—high blood pressure, overweight, dangerously high cholesterol. It was time for action. With determined dedication, she enrolled in a nearby live-in health center. She must get well! And 25 days later she felt like a new woman. Hers was the big success story. Her radiant face and her fit, healthy body were impressive testimonials. For two years she was Exhibit A for anyone interested in healthful lifestyle changes.

Then came the fall. A family crisis took her away from home for an extended period. Stress, anxiety, and weariness took their toll. Her routines were disrupted and her new habits neglected. An inner voice called her from time to time, and promises were made, broken, remade, and broken again. As her goals receded, so did her motivation. Weeks melted into months, then years.

On the golf course one afternoon Angie took a hard swing at a small ball that seemed to symbolize her mounting frustration. A sudden blinding pain landed her back in bed. It was like a flashback to four years earlier. The weight was back, the blood pressure up. And golf, her cherished hobby, was now a literal pain. How could she have let this happen? The realization was a bitter pill. So this was Exhibit A! She'd let everyone down. The pain of humiliation overshadowed her physical suffering. Mrs. Perfect wasn't perfect after all.

She would have to admit it—to herself and to others.

So Angie came back to the health center. She resumed the routine, the walks, the lectures, the food, and the treatments. Once again she got better. During our consultations I encouraged her to be less perfectionistic and more realistic. "You must stop being so obsessed with doing everything 100 percent," I told her. "When you do that, you set yourself up for failure. No one can measure up to such high standards all the time." Her new humility and her willingness to try again made her more receptive to our teaching. "After all," I reminded her, "a 10 percent improvement is better than no improvement."

The day came for our last office visit. "I'm a wiser woman now," she told me. "I'm not out for the big win. It's going to be one day at a time." She looked out the window, reflecting on her situation, then turned to me again. "Failure is no big deal, you know. One big binge will no longer defeat me." Her blue eyes softened. "My secret is that I'm

NATURAL REMEDIES	
Nutrition	Water
Exercise	Air
Rest	Temperance
Sunshine	*Trust in Divine Power*

enlisting outside help. I can relate to a God who instructs His followers to forgive each other at least 490 times. [See Matthew 18:21, 22.] I still have a ways to go!"

We hugged and prayed together. It was our last visit, and we would soon part. I walked back to the lodge with her. "Four years ago I went home with only seven of the natural remedies," she mused. "This time I'm taking the eighth one home, too: trust in divine power. That's the one that will make all the difference."

Part VII

THE SPIRITUAL CONNECTION

Desperation Station
Miracles

Several years ago, during a "manipulation," I experienced excruciating pain, passed out, and awoke with severe neck pain and a loud buzzing sound in my head. The buzzing continued nonstop for two years—24 hours a day, seven days a week. I had to keep the radio or some other kind of noise going much of the time to try to drown out the loud continuous sound. I often felt that I couldn't endure it, that I'd go out of my mind.

During that time I spent thousands of dollars on specialists, X-rays, CAT scans, angiograms—anything that might lead to relief. Finally I was advised to enter the pain clinic at the University of California at Davis Medical Center to learn to live with the condition. I received the application and a questionnaire of more than 900 questions. I looked at that endless list of questions and thought about the time and expense ahead. And for what? My courage failed, and I wept in discouragement.

Then the phone rang. It was my daughter. When I explained my plight, she said, "Mom, forget the pain clinic and go to that live-in health center near where you live."

So I did. When I got there and explained my situation to the doctor, I told her this was my last hope, truly, my desperation station. I could see immediately that I must have said the wrong thing. She became very distressed and tactfully tried to explain to me that their lifestyle program did not treat things such as I had. She told me that all they could do for me was to put me on an optimal general health program and ask the Lord's blessing. I told her that was OK with me. Whatever happened, I would accept the consequences. If healing came, I would be grateful. If it didn't, then with God's help I would live with it.

I plunged into every detail of the program, 100 percent. I attended the classes, ate the food, walked the trails, worked in the garden, and took my treatments. And the problem continued, unabated. But I wasn't discouraged. I loved everything. I knew the staff was praying for me, and the other patients prayed for me too. Healed or not, I was determined to make this a mountaintop experience in my life.

On the eighth day, after my regular physical therapy treatment, it seemed that the noise was decreasing, but I had to rush up to hydrotherapy and didn't think too much about it. As I lay on the hydro table receiving my water treatment, I realized the noise had changed—I could barely hear it. Also, the neck pain was gone. But I was cautious at first, a bit fearful that perhaps it was only a temporary phenomenon.

Within the hour, though, I was convinced that a miracle had happened. And there was rejoicing and praising the Lord and dancing over the trails of the Sierra Nevadas such as I envisioned David must have done as he brought the ark of the covenant back to

Jerusalem! (2 Samuel 6:14, 15).

More than three years have passed since that day. I remain free of the noise, the pressure, and the neck pain. I continue to practice the health principles the Lord gave me through the health center. Since God chose to heal me in this way, I'm dedicated to continuing this lifestyle for life.

I should tell you that my health and energy are better now than at any time in my life. On a recent 11-mile trek into Yosemite National Park, a group of young people wanted a picture of "this 74-year-old white-haired mountaineer."

"When I get old," one girl told me, "I want to be like you."

Every day is a joy to me, and I cannot praise and thank God enough. I want to share this story with the whole world.

Beating Burnout
Stress

My friend kept urging me to take some time off and go to a live-in health program in California, but I kept resisting. I'll admit I was prejudiced. Extremists, I suspected. Maybe even fanatical. Certainly legalistic. A bunch of health nuts, I was sure.

"Why not give it a try?" he urged. "What do you have to lose?"

I guess I didn't have much to lose. I felt lousy and

woke up tired. I was stressed, weary, and depressed. I was losing interest in life, a situation that was entirely out of character for me. I am a pastor; I've been a missionary, and I've been promoted to a church leadership position that takes me all over the world. I also edit an important religious magazine for my church. All my life I've worked hard and thrived on it. I had certainly never been bored. I loved my work. It had always been challenging, exciting, and fulfilling.

So what was the matter now? Perhaps I was burned out. Maybe this was the signal, the way it felt when it was time to quit. My friend knew I was giving serious thought to retirement. After all, I was nearly 65 years old. My friend also knew that I hated the thought of quitting.

I struggled on for another three months. But I was definitely over the hill and going down the other side. Vacations didn't help, and hospital admission was out of the question. But what could a health center do for me? My wife and I had always been careful about our health. I had even taught health principles in my ministry. We were vegetarians. I was sure I knew it all. True, I was quite a bit overweight and had an understandable human weakness for desserts, but was that enough to bring a man down? Finally, though, I gave in and took a month off to see what would happen.

When I arrived from Washington, D.C., it was like stepping into another world. The place was tucked into the foothills of the Sierra Nevadas, surrounded by tall pines, fresh air, and warm sunshine. Suddenly freed from the pressures of my work, I felt the stress begin melting away. The staff was friendly, caring, dedicated, and talented. Everything seemed perfect.

The first meal, however, was a shocker and restored my suspicions. I felt like King Nebuchadnezzar of Daniel's day, who, after losing his reason, began eating grass! Was it necessary for food to be so tasteless? The food was all—and I mean *all*—unrefined. Because even orange and apple juices are refined, we were taught to get our juice in its natural form—by eating the whole fruit. The cooks use no animal products, such as milk, cheese, or eggs. They use little salt and no extracted oils, grease, or refined sugars in preparing the food.

After about a week I decided they must have changed cooks, because the food tasted decidedly better. And by the end of my stay I was actually relishing the plain, unadulterated food. It was a real eye-opener to realize how far I, a conscientious, health-minded person, had strayed from eating natural food, simply prepared.

MAYBE THIS WAS THE SIGNAL, THE WAY IT FELT WHEN IT WAS TIME TO QUIT.

Exercise was the next important factor to impact us newcomers. Most of us know we need exercise, but few of us really understand the enormous difference it can make in our health and well-being. I was soon hiking more than five miles a day in the exhilarating mountain atmosphere.

Many other benefits came my way as well, such as relaxing massage and water treatments, increased time to study God's Word, the morning devotionals, and the beautiful prayers of persons ministering to us.

Although medicines were given when needed, this health center is based on eight natural health principles: healthful food, active exercise, liberal use of water, exposure to sunshine and fresh air, temperance (avoidance of all harmful substances, such as cigarettes, alcohol, caffeine, and some drugs), adequate rest—all on a foundation of faith, a living trust in the God who created us.

The genius of this program is found in the marvelous blending together of every element that touches our lives. The focus was not only to revive us but to teach us a way of life we could take home and continue to live for the rest of our lives. To that end we were gently instructed in the whys and hows of a healthy lifestyle, with practical cooking demonstrations and scientific yet understandable lectures by health professionals.

The results were not only good—they were astounding! After only two weeks I felt like a new man. By the fourth week I was my old self again—energetic, optimistic, creative, and on fire. I could hardly wait to get back to my work.

∞

It's been nearly 10 years, and I've retained most of my gains. I'm 32 pounds lighter, and I walk three to five miles a day. And I, admittedly the weakest of the weak when it comes to food, have been able to make some major changes. For one thing, I have cut out dairy products. Besides lowering my dangerously high cholesterol level and helping me to lose weight, this change has relieved me of the stuffed-up nose I had suffered from for years. What a joy to breathe freely once more and to feel good every new day!

Looking back, I view that time as a beautiful spiritual experience—an opportunity to learn how God meant us to live. The program consists of many threads tightly woven into a pattern of beauty. Threads of prayer, encouragement, scientific evidence, practice, fellowship, and study are all woven together into the healing process.

Retire? Don't be ridiculous! Yes, I have retired, but only from a full-time salary. I am still going strong, working for a religious television program, *It Is Written*. I would rather die with my boots on. But until then I plan to concentrate on doing what I love most—writing and preaching.

NOTE: Unfortunately, a few months after giving me this story, Pastor Spangler, on his way to a preaching appointment, was instantly killed in a freeway accident. It did fulfill his wish, however—he "went out with his boots on."

∽

Stress has come to be linked with almost every medical problem we have these days—heart attacks, hypertension, heart disease, ulcers, colitis, headaches, backaches, asthma, nervous breakdowns, even cancer. Yet too little stress can invite disease as well, causing fatigue, boredom, restlessness, dissatisfaction, and depression. The challenge is to find a middle road between the two extremes.

The pace of modern life has thrown us into a kind of time warp. We are constantly urged to go now, see now, buy now, enjoy now. After all, as the ads tell us, we have only one chance in life, and we'd better grab all we can.

However, after a few years of grabbing, getting, going, seeing, and buying, we begin to feel battered and disappointed. The inevitable *pay later* comes along—burnout, debts, poor health, depression, and loss of interest in life. It's a vicious cycle that has trapped many well-meaning men and women.

Health has been called the ability to adapt to life's stresses. If this is so, healthy people must find ways to pace themselves by keeping their stress in positive balance.

Much of life does give us a choice. Don't procrastinate! Choose to enjoy life as it goes by. Praise the sunshine and the rain. Smell the flowers, return the smiles, play with children. This approach to life costs little and avoids hangovers. It exacts no *pay later* debt. Instead, it pays generous dividends.

HOW TO MANAGE STRESS

- *Regular active exercise* for at least 30 minutes a day. Exercise produces endorphins, the *feel good* hormones that protect the body against stress. Sunshine and fresh air also produce endorphins, so outdoor exercise is doubly beneficial.

- *A simple, plant-food-centered diet.* The body easily handles such a diet. The result is increased energy, efficiency, and endurance.

- *No cigarettes, alcohol, caffeine, or other harmful drugs.* These substances all chalk up substantial *pay later* debts, often beginning the next day.

- *Adequate rest.* This includes a good night's sleep and regular times for relaxation and recreation.

- *Liberal use of water—inside and out.* Drink enough water to keep the urine pale (six to eight glasses a day). A hot and cold shower each morning starts your day off right.

- *Stable life anchors.* A religious faith, a loving home, a job that makes you feel worthwhile, inspiring friends, a purpose for living—these are all vaccines against stress.

- *A positive mental attitude.* Picture a very cranky man walking to work in the pouring rain, cursing all the way. What is going on inside this man? Now picture three delighted children playing in the same rain. What is going on inside these children? Who has the most stress? The difference is not in the circumstances but in the attitude toward those circumstances.

Mind Power

Immune System

I don't drink coffee. I don't even know how to make it. But one particular night I had a special need. I was working late, trying to finish an important project, and I was nearly overwhelmed by sleepiness. Remembering that my secretary keeps a jar of instant coffee in her desk, I added several tablespoons of that brown chunky powder to a cup of cold water, gulped it down, and waited.

Within 10 minutes I felt energized. (Yes, caffeine mobilizes blood sugar.) Then came heightened alertness. (Yes, it also stimulates the nervous system.) I rushed to the bathroom, confirming that caffeine is also a diuretic. The boost lasted the three hours I needed to finish the project. The next morning I confessed to my secretary. She listened and began to smile.

"I'm glad my coffee helped," she said. "But didn't you notice? It was *decaffeinated!*"

I realized I had been a victim of what is called the placebo effect. Because I fully expected it to work, it did work. The placebo effect is commonly used to test new medicines. One group of test subjects is given the real thing, while another group receives the look-alike. Surprisingly, placebo subjects often report the same results as those who receive the actual medication. (Of course, the placebo group doesn't have to cope with the medication's side effects.)

For a long time scientists didn't believe there was a direct link between emotion and disease, because they couldn't take one particular emotion, such as anger, and relate it to a specific disease, such as a heart attack. But nowadays they can measure the body's immune response to specific stresses.

The body's immune system can be described as millions of *fighting units,* circulating in the blood-stream. These consist of different types of *soldiers* (blood cells), each group having its own specific function. *Central control* can order out new *units* when disease invades the body. During times of peace the numbers are reduced, and the *fighters* become patrols. This is a simplified explanation of the immune system.

EVERY DAY WE ENCOUNTER HUNDREDS OF GERMS THAT COULD MAKE US SICK OR EVEN KILL US.

It appears that a healthful diet, physical fitness, and positive emotional states can stimulate and strengthen the body's immune system. On the other hand, illness, drugs, and chronic stress can weaken it.

Scientists report that people in depressed and negative emotional states may be especially vulnerable to diseases affecting the immune system, such as asthma, allergies, rheumatoid arthritis, and cancer. AIDS occurs when the entire immune system has been destroyed.

There is no longer any question that thoughts and emotions do directly influence the mind, which, in turn, can powerfully affect the body. Reports are on record of people who believed they were going to die, and they did, even though no direct cause could be found. This powerful effect of the mind on the body relates directly to the immune system. Every day we encounter hundreds of germs that could make us sick or even kill us. When our immune system is healthy and well, the bad things that attack us are fought off, and our health is preserved.

Scientists are now suggesting that a stable emotional life is as important to good health as more traditional influences, such as improved diet, regular exercise, and the avoidance of alcohol, tobacco, and other drugs.

Positive emotions and sensible health practices, it appears, can stimulate the production of endorphins. These mysterious substances are manufactured by the brain and can produce remarkable feelings of well-being. Apparently they pep up the immune system as well. Endorphins, in other words, help make you feel better while they also help keep you well.

The amazing thing is that these concepts come right out of the Bible. King Solomon advises, "A cheerful heart is good medicine, but a crushed spirit dries up the bones" (Proverbs 17:22, NIV). And Paul adds, "Whatever is true, whatever is noble, whatever is right, whatever is pure, whatever is lovely, whatever is admirable—if anything is excellent or praiseworthy—think about such things" (Philippians 4:8, NIV).

How Much Are You Worth?

Self-esteem

The story is told of a speaker who started off his seminar by holding up a $20 bill. In the room of 200 people he asked, "Who would like this $20 bill?"

Hands started going up.

"I'm going to give this $20 bill to one of you, but first let me do this." He proceeded to crumple the bill into a small wad. "Now who wants it?"

The hands went up again.

"Well," he replied, "what if I do this?" He unfolded the crumpled bill and dropped it on the ground and started to grind it into the floor with his shoe. He picked it up, now all crumpled and dirty. "Anybody want it now?"

All the hands still went up.

"My friends," he said, "you have all learned a valuable lesson. No matter what I do to the money, you still want it, because it has not decreased in value. It is still worth $20. Many times in our lives we are dropped, crumpled, and ground into the dirt by the decisions we make and the circumstances that come our way. We feel as though we are worthless. But no matter what has happened, or what will happen, we never lose our value in God's eyes. Dirty or clean, crumpled or creased, we are still priceless to Him. You see, the

IT TAKES MORE THAN HEALTHY FOOD AND REGULAR EXERCISE TO MAKE LIFE WORTHWHILE.

137

worth of our lives comes not in what we do or who we are—but by Whose we are!"

Deep down most of us harbor feelings of low self-esteem. Although Americans live longer, healthier lives than ever before, surveys show they feel less and less satisfied with their lives. We are increasingly a nation of whiners and hypochondriacs.

"If I could write a prescription for the women of this world," says James Dobson, "I would provide each one of them with a healthy dose of self-esteem and personal worth. I have no doubt that this is their greatest need."

Feelings of worthlessness and low self-esteem are certainly no respecter of persons. They cross lines of gender, race, age, color, and ethnic origin. People today are bombarded with overinflated expectations, grandiose hopes, and unrealistic representations of life. When their dreams fade and their hopes crash, when disappointments pile up, many become disillusioned and discouraged. Other people seem to be doing better than they're doing. They've missed out somehow. Life is passing them by.

Most problems with self-esteem have their roots in childhood. What happens during the first five years pretty much sets children's attitudes for the rest of their lives. Many children grow up feeling unloved, neglected, and unwanted. They are yelled at and otherwise abused. Surrounded with too many negative messages and rules, they often are sullen, rebellious, hostile, and difficult to handle. As teenagers, their feelings of worthlessness intensify. They long to be attractive, to be popular, or even just to be noticed.

Their low level of self-confidence suppresses their talents and their personalities. The result is loneliness, isolation, perhaps bad relationship choices, and often drugs and prostitution.

Most of us honestly admit that we seek a renewing purpose in life, a sense that life matters, that we can contribute something to the world. God knows this. He certainly didn't intend for any of us to suffer from low self-esteem. "I have loved you with an everlasting love," He tells us. "I have drawn you with loving-kindness" (Jeremiah 31:3, NIV). "Cast all your anxiety on him because he cares for you" (1 Peter 5:7, NIV). "You are all [children] of God" (Galatians 3:26, NIV). Jesus Himself, when summing up the two greatest commandments, said that the second was "Love your neighbor as yourself" (Mark 12:30, 31, NIV).

Ultimate self-esteem comes from knowing who we are, why we are here, and where we are going. The Bible answers these questions in a beautiful and meaningful way.

WHO ARE WE?

We are God's unique creation (Genesis 1:27). Among all the billions of people who have been born on our globe, there are no duplicates—not even among identical twins. And that isn't all. We're told that God "knit [us] together in [our] mother's womb" (Psalm 139:13, NIV). He knows when we sit down and get up. He understands our thoughts. Read Psalm 139 for yourself. It spells out God's care, starting as early as our conception.

God also assures us that He is no respecter of persons. "There is neither Jew nor Greek, slave nor free, male nor female, for you are all one in Christ Jesus" (Galatians 3:28. NIV).

And the same God continues to love us unconditionally today. "Are not five sparrows sold for two pennies? Yet not one of them is forgotten by God. Indeed, the very hairs of your head are all numbered. Don't be afraid; you are worth more than many sparrows" (Luke 12:6, 7, NIV).

WHY ARE WE HERE?

To take care of the earth and its people, and to spread the good news of a God who loves all His creation. (See Genesis 1:26; Mark 12:31; 16:15.)

WHERE ARE WE GOING?

Nearly everyone knows God's answer to this one. "For God so loved the world that he gave his one and only Son, that whoever believes in him shall not perish but have eternal life" (John 3:16, NIV).

Jesus told His disciples that His Father's house has many rooms. He would be going there to prepare a place for them, then He would come back to take them home with Him (see John 14:1-3).

It is only when we recognize the value each of us represents to our Creator that we gain true self-esteem. When we love ourselves, when we learn to fully appreciate this life God has given us, we can reach out to others and learn to love them too.

Studies indicate that people who are shown affection are less likely to see a doctor or feel sick. They also report a zest for life, love for work, and a sense that their existence is meaningful. Obviously it takes a lot more than healthy food and regular exercise to make life worthwhile. People need dignity and respect. The need to love and be loved is as essential to health and well-being as fresh air and clean water.

Too many people base their self-esteem on what other people think of them. But people's opinions are fickle, unstable, and certainly not worth depending on.

Christ never passed by a human being as worthless, and we can't either. With a restored sense of self-worth, we become willing to take risks. And taking risks in loving others is what life is all about.

"Dear friends, let us love one another, for love comes from God. . . . Since God so loved us, we also ought to love one another." "Let us not love with words or tongue but with actions" (1 John 4:7-11; 3:18, NIV).

Thank God for Cancer!
Finding God

"What? You welcomed cancer?" I thought I'd heard everything, but this was a new one. "But why? After AIDS, cancer is the most dreaded disease in the world!"

Carol gave it to me straight. "I've lived a very self-destructive lifestyle. For years I haven't cared about my health. I've smoked since my early teens, and I drank heavily for a long time. My life seemed so empty and worthless that I began to wish I could die. When the doctors told me after lung surgery that they'd found cancer, I actually felt relief. The sooner I died, the better. I couldn't think of anything I wanted to live for."

OFTEN THE TEST OF COURAGE IS NOT TO DIE, BUT TO LIVE.

"So why are you here?" I asked. Carol wasn't shy about sharing her reasons. Here's her story:

I was raised a strict Roman Catholic and spent several years in a convent. But I was rebellious, and when my 23-year-old brother gave me a cigarette, I not only smoked it, I continued to smoke. I also began dating, but I mostly sat around smoking with the boys. I was 14 years old. When I was 18 I married a struggling young medical student. I was a talented singer and got a job singing with the St. Louis metropolitan opera for four years. My earnings helped put my husband through medical school.

As time went by, problems mounted, and my husband began drinking. When our marriage began deteriorating, I followed his example. By the time I was 38 I was a divorced woman with three children to finish raising. I held various jobs—secretary, photographer, and bar owner.

Two years later I married an engineer. He was a good provider, and I had everything I needed materially. But I couldn't seem to find myself, to find my place in life. My husband's dominant nature and overprotectiveness smothered me. I longed for some recognition in life, besides just being a servant to John.

My alcoholism worsened to the point that I had a seizure five years ago and spent three days in a coma. I quit drinking, not because I wanted to live, but because as long as I had to live, I didn't want to be crippled or lose my mind.

But my smoking increased. I often sat up far into the night, smoking cigarettes and drinking coffee. I developed a chronically worsening case of bronchitis, an ulcer, and finally angina pains. My blood pressure went sky-high, and I had a small stroke. Despite all of this, I never seriously tried to stop smoking. Not even after my lung cancer surgery. I just didn't care.

My family was pretty upset by this time, but they felt helpless because they didn't know what to do for me. One of my husband's employees had gone through one of your programs here at the health center. He told me I could find a whole new way of life at this place. By that time I was so depressed and sick that I actually began to want help. When my husband offered to come with me, I decided to come. But I'm scared. I have no idea what I'm getting into.

∞

At first Carol told me she wanted only to cut down her smoking. But by the second day she felt sufficiently encouraged and supported to make the break—cold turkey. The next five days were full of misery. Constant nausea, punctuated by vomiting, reactivated her ulcer. Her stomach hurt terribly. The headaches didn't let up. Her blood pressure reached 230/100. But she didn't quit; she stuck it out. Here is how she described the experience:

"The staff stayed right with me. I was tenderly and lovingly cared for. I had lots of water treatments, consisting of hot packs, whirlpool, and cooling baths. They pushed fluids. I must have had 20 cups of water a day. Gradually the withdrawal symptoms subsided. By the sixth day my blood pressure was back to normal, and I slept nine hours straight for the first time in five years!"

As the nicotine and carbon monoxide washed out of her system, more oxygenated blood reached her heart, and the angina faded. Before she left she was walking five miles without pain. She was able to stop all six of her medicines.

"It's hard to realize how miserable and depressed I was just three weeks ago," Carol told me. "My life is so different now. The craving for cigarettes is gone. My whole outlook has changed. My husband is delighted! What's surprising," she continued, "is that the most valuable thing I found here is not freedom from my smoking habit or the ability to hike trails without angina pain. It is reconnecting with a God who cares for me and who wants me to be whole, both physically and spiritually. I am hopeful now. I have a reason to live. I have finally found the way to fill that empty void in my life. Yes, I can honestly say I thank God for my cancer, not because I want to die, but because it led me to a new life with Him."

The Key to Peace

Forgiveness

A wealthy, well-educated, yet deeply depressed woman came to me for counseling. She complained of recurrent headaches, ulcers, and obesity. "I just can't get rid of this weight. I'm bloated with fat," she said as the tears began to flow.

Then, through her tears, she wailed, "He did this to me!" Her husband, a respected politician, had had an affair. "I hate him for it, and I hate the woman even more. They've ruined my life."

Even though the affair had occurred 11 years before, the woman was still obsessed with her bitterness and anger.

"You need to know about the healing option," I tried to explain. "You are allowing the hurts of the past to make a mockery of your life today. A painful memory is a mental wound, and you must let it heal. You must stop picking at the scab. You can't afford to keep an emotional scrapbook of your painful memories, because this is what imprisons you."

As the woman began to understand these principles, she realized how she had actually perpetuated her problems. She had mortgaged her present joy by clinging to her past. She needed to internalize the excellent counsel given years before by the apostle Paul to the Philippians: "There is one thing I have done and will continue to do, and that is to forget things that are in the past and to look ahead toward the spiritual goal held out to us by God" (Philippians 3:13, 14, Clear Word).

The woman finally realized she had to move away from her growth-stifling "poor me, pity me" attitudes and to begin to tackle her problems and learn how to solve them.

A PAINFUL MEMORY IS A MENTAL WOUND, AND YOU MUST LET IT HEAL. YOU MUST STOP PICKING AT THE SCAB.

"The moment I started to hate that adulterous woman," she reflected, "I became her slave. For 11 years she has had a tyrannical grasp on my mind and my body. *No more!* I know now that I can learn something positive even from the most desperate situation. God can help me forgive. That woman will not steal my joy for even *one more day* of my life."

This world is a university of hard knocks. We owe it to life not to get bitter. Bitterness shrivels the spirit. It causes spiritual atherosclerosis. Just as wrong foods harden our arteries, nurturing the wrong emotions hardens our attitudes. Our difficulties and disappointments can actually help us to grow in insight, in understanding, and in finding new directions for our lives.

A scientist once watched a butterfly struggling to get out of its cocoon. It seemed that it simply could not force its way through such a small opening. After watching for a while, he "helped" the butterfly by enlarging the hole with some scissors. The butterfly emerged with a swollen body and shriveled wings. It never flew. The well-intentioned "help" deprived the butterfly of the struggle to get through the small opening that would have forced the fluid from its body into its still-developing wings.

Ernest Hemingway tells the touching story of a great quarrel between a father and his teenage son, Paco. Their relationship shatters, and the son leaves home. The father soon regrets the episode and begins the search for his son. But the city of Madrid is so large, so confusing—the father hasn't a clue where to look. In desperation he decides to put an ad in the paper. "Dear Paco, meet me at 10:00 tomorrow morning in front of the newspaper office. All is forgiven. I love you. Dad." The next morning the father finds 800 Pacos in front of the newspaper office, all searching, all hoping.

Our world is full of hurting, heartbroken people, people who have been mistreated, neglected, alienated, and victimized; people who are angry, resentful, bitter, lonely, and depressed; fearful and guilt-ridden people consumed by hatred and self-pity. But our world is also full of people longing for love, acceptance, compassion, and forgiveness; for someone to care; for spiritual comfort and peace of mind. At best we have a limited number of days in our lives. Isn't each day too precious to be marred by unforgiving thoughts?

People who learn to forgive suffer less anxiety and depression and have greater self-esteem. And they enjoy better health. A wise man said, "If you cannot forgive, you will live lonely, and the wine of life will be soured for you forever."

On a lonely hill, cruel, unfeeling soldiers were driving spikes through the hands and feet of a prisoner, nailing Him to a cross. "Father, forgive them," the prisoner prayed, "for they do not know what they are doing" (Luke 23:34, NIV). The result? A Roman centurion and one of the thieves were forgiven that very day.

Love is more important than being right. Forgiveness opens the heart. Truly, to err is human, to forgive, divine.

> "Hatred is like acid. It does more harm to the container in which it is stored than to the object on which it is poured."—Ann Landers.

The Ultimate Gift

Love

M rs. Hannah's only daughter was raped and murdered by a man who was subsequently put in prison for life. It had been hard enough to lose her husband in a car accident, but now to have her only child so brutally killed was more than she could bear. She hated that man with every fiber and emotion of her being. Every day she prayed that his life would be as miserable as hers.

One day a Gideon (a person who supplies hotels, motels, and other public places with Gideon Bibles) came to her home and asked if she would care to inscribe a Bible for that murderer. Although she had been a religious person, she angrily refused. Surely God would not expect her to do such a thing!

For weeks and months Mrs. Hannah struggled. Her focus had become revenge. Gone were any feelings of joy or personal triumph. Eventually, though, she realized that she too was a prisoner—trapped in her own prison of misery.

IT'S WHAT WE VALUE, NOT WHAT WE HAVE, THAT MAKES US RICH.

In the end Mrs. Hannah knelt down and pleaded with God to forgive her feelings of bitterness and hatred. And when she did, she felt an easing of her burden. In due time she called the Gideon and asked him to bring back that Bible, because now she was ready and willing.

She opened the Bible and wrote, "Mrs. Hannah loves you." When the prisoner read this message, tears flowed down his cheeks. He had grown up an orphan. Never had anyone told him that he was loved. That one sentence changed his life. He became a prison chaplain and spent the rest of his life ministering to other prisoners.

And on that very day when Mrs. Hannah penned those words her own self-imposed sentence of "life imprisonment" was commuted. The bitter, hateful Mrs. Hannah had died. The new Mrs. Hannah stepped outside, took a deep breath of fresh spring air, felt the sunshine on her face, noticed the flowers—and sang for joy. She was free at last!

The Root of Health

Trust in Divine Power

I consider trust in divine power to be the most important factor necessary for true healing. A for-real relationship with the true God, our Creator, is never optional to health—it is the very root of health. Trust in God has profound effects on both the physical mechanisms of the body and the workings of the mind.

For example, I believe that joyful trust in God enables Him to increase and harmonize beneficial neurohormones, such as the endorphins and possibly serotonin. Research studies indicate that the rise of such levels benefits one's total health. These hormones have a great calming, relaxing influence, bringing deeper restorative sleep, reducing depression, strengthening the immune system, controlling pain, and stabilizing one's emotions. All of these factors are crucial to healing of any kind.

TRUST IN DIVINE POWER MEANS GETTING TO KNOW GOD WELL ENOUGH TO TRUST HIM FOR PRESENT AND FUTURE WELL-BEING.

Without trust in God, the mind is often plagued with fears, doubts, and anger. These stress factors are associated with rising adrenaline and corticoid levels that relate to tension, a rise in blood pressure, increased fatigue, and insomnia, and they can even hinder the effectiveness of medications.

Many people can—and do—find successful healing on a purely physical level. But without a trusting

150

relationship with the God from whom the healing truly comes, all the other measures give only a temporary solution to the body's needs. But when trust is added, God can do so much more. He can multiply the benefits received from other remedies, and He can extend healing into all dimensions—the physical, mental, emotional, and spiritual. This is why I say that genuine health comes from one's relationship with the true God.

What does trust in divine power mean? Simply that people open their minds and hearts to God's love and mercy and allow His healing power to flow into their lives. It means getting to know God well enough to trust Him for present and future well-being.

This is not a radical or new idea! Our health, happiness, longevity, and self-esteem, as well as our family, our friends and associates, and our spiritual life are interrelated and interdependent.

The Bible says that "a merry heart doeth good like a medicine: but a broken spirit drieth the bones" (Proverbs 17:22). Health isn't just eating and drinking and exercising. It is also "righteousness, peace, and joy in the Holy Spirit" (Romans 14:17, NIV).

—Sang Lee, M.D.

Abstracted from an article (used with permission)

Part VIII

CODA

To win the battle against the lifestyle-related diseases we must adopt a simpler, more natural way of eating. We need to eat a variety of plant food the way it grows, either raw or prepared with very little fat, oil, sugar, or salt. We also must avoid refined foods such as white bread and white rice, white sugar, as well as most fast foods.

Animal foods are devoid of fiber, are too high in protein, and contain a lot of fat and cholesterol. It is therefore best to drastically restrict all meat, chicken, fish, cheese, and ice cream, and use nonfat dairy food as much as possible.

The good news is that this kind of diet will both prevent many of these diseases and help heal those already present. In addition, we will enjoy better health,

---

THE PREVENTIVE (OPTIMAL) DIET

This diet will prevent many of today's lifestyle diseases. Notice how it compares with the average American (Western) diet:

	Western Diet/Day	*Preventive Diet/Day*
Fats and oils	35-40 percent of calories	15-20 percent of calories
Sugar	35 teaspoons	< 10 teaspoons
Cholesterol	400 milligrams	< 50 milligrams
Salt	10-15 grams	< 5 grams
Fiber	10 grams	40-50 grams

THE REVERSAL DIET

The Reversal Diet is for those who already have an advanced case of one or more of the lifestyle diseases. We know that a "stricter" limitation of fat and cholesterol intake will, over time, result in a gradual unplugging of clogged arteries. Improved circulation of the blood allows affected areas to start healing and can sometimes bring about a reversal of the illness. Here is how the Reversal Diet compares to the Preventive Diet.

	Preventive Diet/Day	Reversal Diet/Day
Fats and oils	15-20 percent of calories	10-15 percent of calories
Sugar	< 10 teaspoons	< 10 teaspoons
Cholesterol	< 50 milligrams	0 milligrams
Salt	< 5 grams	< 5 grams
Fiber	40-50 grams	40-50 grams

have more energy, and even reduce our grocery bills.

The menus for the Reversal Diet are essentially the same as for the Preventive (Optimal) Diet except that it is advisable to completely avoid any foods of animal origin and all visible fats, and to use only non-fat dressings for salads.

SAMPLE MENU: PREVENTIVE (OPTIMAL) DIET

Breakfast
- Cooked cereal (seven-grain cereal, rolled oats, millet, brown rice, rolled rye, wheat flakes, cracked wheat) or cold cereal (shredded wheat, Grapenuts, Weetabix, Nutri-Grain) with soymilk and sliced banana, berries, or other fresh fruit.
- Citrus fruit: orange, grapefruit. (Eat the fruit rather than drinking the juice.)
- Two slices whole-grain wheat toast with

mashed banana, topped with pineapple ring or slice of kiwi fruit.

- Some nuts and seeds (if overweight, use only sparingly).
- Herbal tea.

Lunch

- Two whole-wheat pita (pocket) breads, stuffed with lettuce, sprouts, cucumbers, tomatoes, radishes, and some low-fat cottage cheese or mashed beans.
- Split-pea soup with pearl barley or rice.
- Fresh fruit, such as papaya, pear, apple.

Dinner

- Whole-wheat spaghetti with tomato sauce.
- A cooked vegetable, such as zucchini.
- Tossed salad with low-calorie Italian dressing.
- Two slices bread with garbanzo or other bean spread.
- For dessert: baked apple, stuffed with dates and walnuts.

If snack is needed: fresh fruit, crisp raw vegetables.

LIVE FOR HEALTH!

THE RIGHT WEIGHT

How can I tell if I'm *fit* or *fat?*

By definition, obese means being 20 percent or more above one's ideal weight. A person with an ideal weight of 120 pounds would be obese at 144 pounds or more. Overweight, on the other hand, means being 10 to 19 percent above one's ideal weight. Our hypothetical person with an ideal weight of 120 pounds would be overweight at 132 to 143 pounds.

How is "ideal" weight determined?

Large life insurance companies have discovered that certain ideal weight-to-height relationships correlate well with optimum life expectancy. (See table below.)

IDEAL WEIGHTS FOR ADULTS ACCORDING TO FRAME

Metropolitan Life Insurance Height/Weight Table (1959)* (Weight in lbs.)[†]

	MEN				WOMEN		
Height[‡]	Small Frame	Medium Frame	Large Frame	Height[‡]	Small Frame	Medium Frame	Large Frame
5'2"	115-123	121-133	129-144	4'10"	96-104	101-113	109-125
5'4"	121-129	127-139	135-152	5'0"	102-110	107-119	115-131
5'6"	128-137	134-147	142-161	5'2"	108-116	113-126	121-138
5'8"	136-145	142-156	151-170	5'4"	114-123	120-135	129-146
5'10"	144-154	150-165	159-179	5'6"	122-131	128-143	137-154
6'0"	152-162	158-175	168-189	5'8"	130-140	136-151	145-163
6'2"	160-171	167-185	178-199	5'10"	138-148	144-159	153-173
6'4"	168-179	177-195	187-209				

*Many established researchers consider the 1959 table of the Metropolitan Life Insurance Company more consistent with good health than the revised 1983 table with its higher values.
[†]Includes one pound for ordinary indoor clothing.
[‡]No Shoes

How is bone size calculated?

In general, a wrist measurement for women of five and one-quarter inches or less is considered small-boned. Between five and one-quarter to six inches is medium; and more than six inches is large. For men, anything under six inches is small, and anything over seven inches is large.

EAT FOR HEALTH!
Basic Guidelines for a Lifetime of Good Eating

EAT LESS:

 Visible fats and oils

Strictly limit fatty meats, cooking and salad oils, sauces, dressings, and shortening. Use margarine very sparingly, and nuts in small amounts. Avoid frying; sauté instead with a little water in nonstick pans.

 Sugars

Limit sugar, honey, molasses, syrups, pies, cakes, pastries, candy, cookies, soft drinks, and sugar-rich desserts—such as pudding and ice cream. Save these foods for special occasions.

 Foods containing cholesterol

Strictly limit meat, sausages, egg yolks, and liver. Limit dairy products, if used, to low-fat cheeses and nonfat milk products. If you eat fish and poultry, use them sparingly.

 Salt

Use mineral salt during cooking. Banish the salt shaker. Strictly limit highly salty products, such as pickles, crackers, soy sauce, salted popcorn, nuts, chips, pretzels, and garlic salt.

 Alcohol

Avoid alcohol in all forms, as well as caffeinated beverages such as coffee, colas, and black tea.

Whole grains
Freely use brown rice, millet, barley, corn, wheat, and rye. Also eat freely of whole-grain products, such as breads, pastas, shredded wheat, and tortillas.

Tubers and legumes
Freely use all kinds of white potatoes, sweet potatoes, and yams (without high-fat toppings). Enjoy peas, lentils, chickpeas, and beans of every kind.

Fruits and vegetables
East several fresh whole fruits every day. Limit fiber-poor fruit juices and fruits canned in syrup. Eat a variety of vegetables daily. Enjoy fresh salads with low-calorie, low-salt dressings.

Water
Drink six to eight glasses of water a day. Vary the routine with a twist of lemon and occasional herb teas.

Hearty breakfasts
Enjoy hot multigrain cereals, fresh fruit, and whole-wheat toast. Jumpstart your day.

Basic Guidelines for a Lifetime of Healthful Living

A checklist for making your NEW START:

Nutrition

- Nourish your body with healthful, full-fiber, nutrient-rich foods.
- Increasingly move toward a totally vegetarian lifestyle.
- Enhance digestion by breaking the snack habit.
- Schedule regular mealtimes, four to five hours apart.
- Eat larger breakfasts and smaller evening meals.

Exercise

- Strengthen your body and increase your enjoyment of life with daily active exercise, outdoors if possible.
- Aim for at least 30 minutes of exercise daily. Walking is the safest exercise, and one of the best. Alternate with strength training.
- Physical exercise reduces stress, combats depression, restores energy, improves sleep, and strengthens bones.

Water

- Rinse out and refresh your insides by drinking a glass or two of water on arising.
- Come alive with an alternating hot and cold shower in the morning.
- Lighten your body's metabolic load and increase circulation by drinking plenty of water— at least eight glasses per day.

Sunshine

- Pull back the drapes! Fill your home with sunshine! It will lift your spirits, brighten your day, and improve your health.

- Spend at least a few minutes outdoors every day.

Temperance

- Live a balanced life. Make time for work, play, rest, exercise, and hobbies.
- Nurture relationships and spiritual growth.
- Protect your body from harmful substances, such as tobacco, alcohol, caffeine, and most drugs.

Air

- Air out your house daily. Sleep in a room with good ventilation.
- Keep your lungs healthy by taking frequent deep breaths. Walk outdoors when possible.
- Fill your house with green plants that absorb carbon dioxide and increase oxygen.

Rest

- Reserve seven to eight hours a night for rest and sleep. The body needs this time to repair and restore the damage of daily wear and tear.
- Go to bed early enough to wake up feeling refreshed.
- Devote time to a change of pace. Go on a picnic, plant a garden, pursue a hobby, take relaxing, enjoyable vacations, take in a concert, attend church.

Trust

- A life of quality and fulfillment includes spiritual growth and development.
- Love, faith, trust, and hope are health-enhancing. And they bring rewards that endure.
- Trust in God augments all healing—physical, mental, emotional, and spiritual.